# Nurses!
# Test Yourself in
# Non-medical
# Prescribing

## Noel Harris and Diane Shearer

Open University Press

Open University Press
McGraw-Hill Education
McGraw-Hill House

Shoppenhangers Road
Maidenhead
Berkshire
England
SL6 2QL

email: enquiries@openup.co.uk
world wide web: www.openup.co.uk

and Two Penn Plaza, New York, NY 10121-2289, USA

First published 2013

Copyright © Noel Harris and Diane Shearer, 2013

A catalogue record of this book is available from the British Library

ISBN-13: 978-0-33-524499-7 (pb)
ISBN-10: 0-33-524499-8 (pb)
eISBN: 978-0-33-524500-0

Library of Congress Cataloging-in-Publication Data
CIP data applied for

Typesetting and e-book compilations by
RefineCatch Limited, Bungay, Suffolk
Printed in Great Britain by CPI Group (UK) Ltd, Croydon, CRO 4YY.

# Contents

# Acknowledgements

We would like to thank Rachel Crookes for encouraging us to collaborate together. We also would like to thank Alex Clabburn, Abbie Jones, and the staff at McGraw-Hill – Open University Press for their patience and support in the process of writing this book. We wish to thank our colleagues and family who have provided good advice and help at important times.

Diane would like to dedicate this book to her parents Barbara and Percy Beales for their continuous love, support, and encouragement.

# About the authors

Dr Noel Harris is a senior lecturer in pharmacology in the School of Health at the University of Northampton, where he teaches science subjects, including biochemistry, physiology, and neuroscience to life science students, as well as pharmacology to nursing and allied health professionals. He has been involved in the teaching of non-medical prescribing courses since 2005.

Diane Shearer is a senior lecturer in the Faculty of Health, Social Care and Education at Anglia Ruskin University where she teaches autonomous practice, advanced clinical skills, and prescribing to nurses, doctors, and allied health professionals. She is also a practising advanced nurse practitioner and current prescriber and has been involved in the provision of non-medical prescribing courses since 2006. She is also currently undertaking doctoral studies looking at multidisciplinary education in prescribing and the reduction of prescribing errors.

# Using this book

Welcome to *Nurses! Test yourself in Non-medical Prescribing.* We hope you will find this an invaluable tool throughout your prescribing courses!

This book is designed to be used as a revision aid that you can use with other textbooks to help you learn the many aspects of prescribing. Each chapter is designed for stand-alone revision, meaning that you need not read from the beginning to benefit from the book. You can dip in and out of the different topics to suit your individual needs.

Every chapter begins with a brief introduction and may point you to to some of the useful resources available to underpin your learning. The chapter progresses, providing you with different types of questions that help you test your knowledge of the area. These are:

- *True or False*: identify if the statement is true or false
- *Multiple Choice*: identify which of 4 answers is/are correct
- *Labelling Exercise*: identify the different elements on the diagram. Sometimes we give you a list of terms to use and sometimes we don't!
- *Fill in the Blanks*: fill in the blanks to complete the statement
- *Match the Terms*: identify which term best matches which statement

The sections have been designed to have some challenging questions in each section. Do not ignore a question type just because you are not examined in that way, because the answer will contain useful information that could easily be examined in an alternative question format.

Answers are provided in each chapter with detailed explanations where appropriate – this is to help you with revision but can also be used as a learning aid.

We have suggested some useful textbooks and other resources that may be used to support your recommended text, they should not replace the core reading for your course.

At the back of the book there is an appendix where you will find a glossary.

We hope that you enjoy using this book and that you find it a convenient and useful tool throughout your studies!

# Guide to useful resources

*Websites*
Association of the British Pharmaceutical industry
www.abpi.org.uk

British National Formulary
www.bnf.org/

Cultural Diversity in Nursing
www.culturaldiversity.org

European Medicines Agency
www.ema.europa.eu

Medicines and Healthcare Products Regulatory Agency
www.mhra.gov.uk

Monthly Index Medical Services (MIMS)
www.mims.co.uk

National Institute for Health and Clinical Excellence
www.nice.org.uk

National Patient Safety Agency
www.npsa.nhs.uk

National Prescribing Centre
www.npc.co.uk

Nurse prescriber forum
www.nurseprescriberforum.co.uk

Nurse prescribing
www.nurseprescribing.com

Nursing and Midwifery Council
www.nmc-uk.org

Skillscascade
www.skillscascade.com

Test and Calc
www.testandcalc.com

Transcultural Nursing
www.culturediversity.org

UK Medicines Information
www.ukmi.nhs.uk

World Health Organization
www.who.int

Yellow Card Scheme
www.yellowcard.mhra.gov.uk

### Books, journals and other resources

*Adherence to Long-Term Therapies: Evidence for Action*
http://apps.who.int/medicinedocs/en/d/Js4883e/5.html
Published by WHO, 2003

*Clinical Decision Making and Judgement in Nursing*
Carl Thompson and Dawn Dowding
Published by Churchill Livingstone, Elsevier, 2001

*Essentials of Pharmacology for Nurses* (2nd Edition)
Paul Barber and Deborah Robinson
Published by McGraw-Hill, 2012

*Fundamentals of Pharmacology: An Applied Approach for Nursing and Health*
Alan Galbraith, Shane Bullock, Elizabeth Manias, Barry Hunt and Ann Richards
Published by Pearson Education, 2007

*Independent and Supplementary Prescribing: An Essential Guide* (2nd Edition)
Molly Courtenay and Matt Griffiths
Published by Cambridge University Press, 2010

*Medicines Adherence: Involving Patients in Decisions about Prescribed Medicines and Supporting Adherence*
Published by NICE, 2011

*Nurse Prescribing* (2nd Edition)
Jennifer L. Humphries and Joyce Green
Published by Palgrave Macmillan, 2002

*Nurse Prescribing: Principles and Practice*
Molly Courtenay and Michele Butler
Published by Greenwich Medical Media, Cambridge University Press, 2000

*Nurses! Test Yourself in Essential Calculation Skills*
K. M. A. Rogers and W. N. Scott
Published by McGraw-Hill, 2011

*Nurses! Test Yourself in Prescribing*
K. M. A. Rogers and W. N. Scott
Published by McGraw-Hill, 2011

*The New Prescriber: An Integrated Approach.*
Joanne Lymn, Dianne Bowskill, Fiona Bath-Hextall and Roger Knaggs
Published by Wiley-Blackwell, 2010

*Transcultural Nursing: Concepts, Theories, Research and Practice* (3rd Edition)
Madeleine Leininger and Marilyn R. McFarland
Published by McGraw-Hill, 2002

# 1 History of prescribing: independent and supplementary

## INTRODUCTION

Non-medical prescribing has taken many years of planning, review, and discussion, and it has been a long-fought and hard-won battle to get to where we are today. From the early days of the 1980s when nurses first began to explore the potential for prescribing certain items such as dressing packs, we are now in the position where nurses are able to prescribe for patients they have assessed and diagnosed independently.

The nursing profession began a claim for jurisdiction of prescribing in 1978 when the Royal College of Nursing (RCN) presented a report proposing that nurses should have authority to prescribe dressings and topical treatments (Jones 1999). It was not until 1986, however, that the Conservative government of the time considered the claim, and a team of health experts and economists were asked to review the provision of community nursing and make recommendations for the future of that provision. The Royal College of Nursing saw this as an ideal opportunity to highlight the arguments for amending legislation to allow nurses to prescribe (Jones and Gough 1997), and following the publication of the report, which was positively received by the government, support was gained from the British Medical Association (BMA) and the Royal Pharmaceutical Society of Great Britain (RPSGB). However, to create a legal framework for nurse prescribing, the 1968 Medicines Act had to be amended. Allowing parliamentary time for the amendments was not, according to Sims and Gardiner (1999), a priority for the government. The amendments were finally made in 1992, fourteen years after the first written report in support of nurse prescribing. Over the following eight years the Labour government embarked upon a programme of prescribing policy growth. Prescribing policies formed part of a wider range of policy developments from the Labour government aimed at increasing the efficiency and cost-effectiveness of the National Health Service (NHS) through modernization.

Since these humble beginnings, nurse prescribing has come of age; from the difficult times of pilot studies, meagre training, 'group protocols', limited formularies and the need (understandably) to prove its worth, to the position we are in today where *nurse independent prescribers* are able to 'prescribe any medicine for any medical condition within their competence, including some controlled drugs for specified medical conditions' (Department of Health 2006).

Understanding the historical perspective and the challenges for implementing non-medical prescribing has, and continues to be, vital in understanding the key part this has played in changing the face of health care and realizing the full potential of nursing as a profession.

**Useful resources**

Courtenay, M. and Butler, M. (2000) *Nurse Prescribing: Principles and Practice.* London: Greenwich Medical.

Humphries, J.L. and Green, J. (eds) (2002) *Nurse Prescribing,* 2nd edn. Basingstoke: Palgrave.

Nursing and Midwifery Council (2006) *Standards of Proficiency for Nurse and Midwife Prescribers.* London: NMC.

## TRUE OR FALSE?

Are the following statements true or false?

**1**  Nurse independent prescribers can write out prescriptions for patients assessed by their nursing colleagues who are not prescribers.

**2**  Prescribing a Prescription Only Medicine (POM) as a supplementary prescriber outside an agreed Clinical Management Plan (CMP) constitutes a criminal offence.

**3**  Dieticians can become supplementary prescribers.

**4**  Midwives can become independent prescribers.

**5**  The National Prescribing Centre (NPC) is the governing body that regulates all prescribers in the UK.

**6**  Once an independent prescriber has qualified, they should no longer work from Patient Group Directions (PGD).

**7**  Pharmacists have always been able to prescribe independently.

**8**  Dentists can authorize supplementary prescribers to prescribe for named patients.

**9** Supplementary prescribers are able to issue private prescriptions.

**10** Nurse independent prescribers are able to give directions to a non-prescriber for the administration of a medicine.

**MULTIPLE CHOICE**

Identify one correct answer for each of the following.

**11** The first document to make recommendations for nurses to take on the role of prescribing was:

a) The Department of Health report on the Review of Prescribing, Supply and Administration of Medicines

b) The Cumberlege Report

c) The First Crown Report

d) The Department of Health NHS Plan

**12** The First Crown report was published in:

a) 1989

b) 1991

c) 1997

d) 1998

**13** Once a nurse has become an independent prescriber, he or she can act as the independent prescriber on a clinical management plan to:

a) other nurses

b) allied health professionals

c) pharmacists only

d) none of the above

**14** Clinical Management Plans need to be updated:

a) yearly

b) every 6 months

c) every 3 months

d) monthly

**15** Supplementary prescribing is most useful for:

a)  long-term conditions

b)  family planning services

c)  out-of-hours services

d)  sexual health clinics

**16** Who is responsible and liable for the actions of supplementary prescribers?

a)  the supplementary prescriber alone

b)  the supplementary prescriber and their employer (through vicarious liability)

c)  the independent prescriber

d)  all of the above

**17** Nurse independent prescribers can prescribe unlicensed medicines only:

a)  by means of a Clinical Management Plan

b)  provided they are competent and take responsibility to do so

c)  with support from their manager

d)  provided a medical practitioner deems them competent and it is within their area of practice and in the best interests of the patient

**18** Nurse independent prescribers can prescribe:

a)  anything from the British National Formulary (BNF) including controlled drugs

b)  anything from the BNF including controlled drugs for palliative care only

c)  anything from the BNF including some controlled drugs for specific indications

d)  anything from the BNF including a limited list of controlled drugs for any indications

**19** All non-medical prescribers must be able to demonstrate recognition of the unique differences between neonates, children and young people:

    a) this applies to *all* independent and supplementary prescribers *only* if they work with children in their area of practice

    b) this *only* applies to nurses

    c) this *only* applies to independent prescribers

    d) this applies to *all* independent and supplementary prescribers

**20** The two important pieces of legislation that cover the sale, use and production of medicines including prescribing rights are:

    a) the Medicines Act 1968 and the Prescription Only Medicines (Human Use) Order 1997

    b) the two Crown Reports

    c) the Medicines Act 1968 and the Cumberlege Report

    d) the Prescription Only Medicines (Human Use) Order 1997 and the First Crown Report

**MATCH THE TERMS**

Match each term with the correct description.

A. DMP

B. HCPC

C. V300 Prescriber

D. OSCE

E. PGD

F. PACT

G. GPhC

**21** Practical or simulated examination used as part of the assessment process for those wishing to qualify as independent prescribers.

**22** Data collected centrally to indicate prescribing patterns nationally and locally.

**23** A doctor who acts as a supervisor for a non-medical prescriber undergoing training.

**24** Regulatory body for allied health professionals.

**25** A written direction for the supply and administration of prescription-only medicines to certain patient groups.

**26** Nurse qualified as both an independent and supplementary prescriber.

**27** Regulatory body for pharmacists.

## FILL IN THE BLANKS

Fill in the blanks in each statement using the options in the box.
*Not all of them are required, so choose carefully!*

| | |
|---|---|
| particular | 1957 |
| Regulatory | independent |
| 1968 | government |
| extended | Parliament |
| formulary | named |
| rectally | supplementary |
| administering | voluntary |
| supply | administration |

**28** The Medicines Act _____ is an Act of _____ of the United Kingdom governing the manufacture and _____ of medicines.

**29** Nurse independent prescribers were formally known as _____ _____ nurse prescribers.

**30** 'Mixing' is defined as 'the combination of two or more medicinal products together for the purposes of _____ them to meet the needs of a _____ patient'.

**31** Supplementary prescribing is a _____ prescribing partnership between an _____ prescriber and a _____ prescriber.

**32** The Medicines and Healthcare Products _____ Agency is a _____ agency.

# ANSWERS

## TRUE OR FALSE?

**1** Nurse independent prescribers can write out prescriptions for patients assessed by their nursing colleagues who are not prescribers.

However, the NMC Standards of Proficiency for Nurse and Midwife Prescribers (2006) state that wherever possible this should be avoided, and go on to say that any nurse or midwife who decides to prescribe for others is accountable for this prescribing.

**2** Prescribing a Prescription Only Medicine (POM) as a supplementary prescriber outside an agreed Clinical Management Plan (CMP) constitutes a criminal offence

This agreement can be in the form of a signature or an electronic record of agreement. The independent prescriber may agree verbally to a CMP, providing that it is confirmed by secure email or fax *before* prescribing occurs and is formally agreed within two working days (NMC 2006).

**3** Dieticians can become supplementary prescribers.

At present, the only professionals who can become supplementary prescribers are nurses, pharmacists, optometrists, physiotherapists, podiatrists, chiropodists, and radiographers.

**4** Midwives can become independent prescribers.

Midwives are governed by the same regulatory body as other nurses (NMC) and the same Standards of Proficiency (NMC 2006), and are thus able to train as independent prescribers.

**5** The National Prescribing Centre (NPC) is the governing body that regulates all prescribers in the UK.

The NPC is an agency that supports the NHS and those who work for it to improve safety, quality, and value for money in the use of medicines for the benefit of patients and the public. The NPC also promotes and supports the continued development of non-medical prescribing through effective policy implementation, advice, and targeted support. The programme aims to increase the recognition and understanding of NMP throughout the NHS in England and works with key audiences to support effective NMP implementation, share examples of practice, and promote activity.

**6**    **Once an independent prescriber has qualified, they should no longer work from Patient Group Directions (PGD).**

There is nothing to stop independent prescribers working from PGDs, although there is little need to once qualified.

**7**    **Pharmacists have always been able to prescribe independently.**

Traditionally, doctors prescribed, nurses administered, and pharmacists dispensed medications. This changed in 2003 when pharmacists became eligible to train as supplementary prescribers. In 2009, the law changed again and pharmacists were then able to train as independent prescribers. Pharmacist independent prescribers can prescribe unlicensed medicines for their patients, on the same basis as doctors and provided that they are competent and take responsibility for doing so.

**8**    **Dentists can authorize supplementary prescribers to prescribe for named patients.**

Dentists are independent prescribers and therefore can authorize a supplementary prescriber to prescribe for a named patient. National Health Service (NHS) regulations define which drugs can be prescribed on the NHS. Until 2004, dentists treating NHS patients were expected to prescribe from the Dental Practitioners Formulary (DPF), a concise list of permissible drugs annexed to the British National Formulary (BNF). The DPF has subsequently been incorporated into the BNF, and is interspersed among drugs that cannot be prescribed by dentists on the NHS. However, a dentist can prescribe any drug from the BNF on private prescription but again must only prescribe within their experience and competence.

**9**    **Supplementary prescribers are able to issue private prescriptions.**

Supplementary and independent prescribers are able to prescribe private prescriptions. For supplementary prescribers, these must be for medications covered by the CMP. For independent prescribers, these can be prescriptions for any medicine within their competence, including some controlled drugs for specified medical conditions.

**10**    **Nurse independent prescribers are able to give directions to a non-prescriber for the administration of a medicine.**

All nurse independent prescribers are able to give directions for the administration of any product he or she is legally allowed to prescribe, i.e. a medicine for a condition within his or her competence. The prescribing nurse needs to be satisfied that the person to whom he or she gives the instructions is competent to administer the medicine concerned.

**MULTIPLE CHOICE**

Correct answers identified in bold italics.

**11** **The first document to make recommendations for nurses to take on the role of prescribing was:**

a) The Department of Health report on the Review of Prescribing, Supply and Administration of Medicines
*b) The Cumberlege Report*
c) The First Crown Report
d) The Department of Health NHS Plan

The Cumberlege Report, *Neighbourhood Nursing: A Focus for Care* (Department of Health and Social Security 1986), recommended that community nurses should be able to prescribe, as part of their everyday nursing care, from a limited list of items.

**12** **The First Crown report was published in:**

*a) 1989* b) 1991 c) 1997 d) 1998

It endorsed nurse prescribing and highlighted the circumstances in which it could occur, and a successful Private Members Bill led to the primary legislation (Medicinal Products: Prescription by Nurses etc. Act 1992) that provided the power for nurses to prescribe.

**13** **Once a nurse has become an independent prescriber, he or she can act as the independent prescriber on a clinical management plan to:**

a) other nurses   b) allied health professionals
c) pharmacists only   *d) none of the above*

This can only be done by a medical practitioner or dentist.

**14** **Clinical Management Plans need to be updated:**

a) yearly.   *b) every 6 months*   c) every 3 months   d) monthly

Generally speaking, clinical management plans should be updated as clinically indicated by response but at least every 6 months to ensure that review of medication is undertaken.

**15** **Supplementary prescribing is most useful for:**

*a)* *long-term conditions*   b) family planning services

c)   out-of-hours services   d) sexual health clinics

Supplementary prescribing can be used for any indication but is generally more useful when review of a condition is required. Thus long-term conditions benefit greatly from this type of prescribing when it is used.

**16** **Who is responsible and liable for the actions of supplementary prescribers?**

a)   the supplementary prescriber alone

*b)* *the supplementary prescriber and their employer (through vicarious liability)*

c)   the independent prescriber

d)   all of the above

When a nurse or midwife is appropriately trained and qualified and prescribes as part of their professional duties with the consent of their employer, the employer is held vicariously liable for their actions. In addition, nurse supplementary prescribers are individually professionally accountable to the Nursing and Midwifery Council (NMC) for this aspect of their practice, as for any other, and must act at all times in accordance with the NMC Code of Professional Conduct.

**17** **Nurse independent prescribers can prescribe unlicensed medicines only:**

a)   by means of a Critical Management Plan

*b)* *provided they are competent and take responsibility to do so*

c)   with support from their manager

d)   provided a medical practitioner deems them competent and it is within their area of practice and in the best interests of the patient

As with all prescribing, nurses should work within the boundaries of the competence in accordance with the NMC guidance.

**18** **Nurse independent prescribers can prescribe:**

*a)* *anything from the British National Formulary (BNF) including controlled drugs*

b)   anything from the BNF including controlled drugs for palliative care only

c)   anything from the BNF including some controlled drugs for specific indications

d)   anything from the BNF including a limited list of controlled drugs for any indications

From April 2012, nurse and pharmacist independent prescribers are allowed to prescribe schedule 2–5 controlled drugs along with all other medications from the BNF, provided they work and prescribe within their clinical competence.

*Note*: Changes to Misuse of Drugs Regulations mean that appropriately qualified nurses and pharmacists will now be able to prescribe controlled drugs like morphine, diamorphine, and prescription strength co-codamol. The changes relating to prescribing and mixing of controlled drugs by nurse and pharmacist independent prescribers also apply to midwives who are registered as nurse independent prescribers.

The agreed changes to the Misuse of Drugs Regulations 2001 relating to nurse and pharmacist independent prescribing of controlled drugs (Misuse of Drugs (Amendment No. 2) (England, Wales and Scotland) Regulations 2012 (Statutory Instrument 2012/973)) came into force on 23 April 2012.

**19** **All non-medical prescribers must be able to demonstrate recognition of the unique differences between neonates, children and young people:**

a) this applies to *all* independent and supplementary prescribers *only* if they work with children in their area of practice

b) this *only* applies to nurses

c) this *only* applies to independent prescribers

d) *this applies to all independent and supplementary prescribers*

**20** **The two important pieces of legislation that cover the sale, use and production of medicines including prescribing rights are:**

a) *the Medicines Act 1968 and the Prescription Only Medicines (Human Use) Order 1997*

b) the two Crown Reports

c) the Medicines Act 1968 and the Cumberlege Report

d) the Prescription Only Medicines (Human Use) Order 1997 and the First Crown Report

 **MATCH THE TERMS**

**21** Practical or simulated examination used as part of the assessment process for those wishing to qualify as independent prescribers.
**D.** OSCE (Objective Structured Clinical Examination)

| **22** | Data collected centrally to indicate prescribing patterns nationally and locally. | **F.** PACT (Prescribing Analysis and Cost) |
| **23** | A doctor who acts as a supervisor for a non-medical prescriber undergoing training. | **A.** DMP (Designated Medical Practitioner) |
| **24** | Regulatory body for allied health professionals. | **B.** HCPC (Health and Care Professions Council) |
| **25** | A written direction for the supply and administration of prescription-only medicines to certain patient groups. | **E.** PGD (Patient Group Direction) |
| **26** | Nurse qualified as both an independent and supplementary prescriber. | **C.** V300 Prescriber |
| **27** | Regulatory body for pharmacists. | **G.** GPhC (General Pharmaceutical Council |

# FILL IN THE BLANKS

**28** **The Medicines Act _1968_ is an Act of _Parliament_ of the United Kingdom governing the manufacture and _supply_ of medicines.**

It also defines three categories: prescription-only medicines (POM), which are available only from a pharmacist if prescribed by an appropriate practitioner; pharmacy medicines (P), available only from a pharmacist but without a prescription; and general sales list (GSL) medicines, which can be bought from a shop without a prescription.

**29** **Nurse independent prescribers were formally known as _extended formulary_ nurse prescribers.**

From 1 May 2006, the former Nurse Prescribers' Extended Formulary was discontinued and qualified nurse independent prescribers, formerly known as extended formulary nurse prescribers, can prescribe any medicine for any medical condition within their competence, including some controlled drugs for specified medical conditions.

**30** **'Mixing' is defined as 'the combination of two or more medicinal products together for the purposes of *administering* them to meet the needs of a *particular* patient'.**

Following the legislative changes in 2009 by the MHRA allowing the mixing of medicines, mixing is defined as above. These changes enable: doctors and dentists, who can already mix medicines themselves, to direct others to mix; nurse and pharmacist independent prescribers to mix medicines themselves and to direct others to mix; supplementary prescribers to mix medicines themselves and to direct others to mix, but only where that preparation forms part of the Clinical Management Plan for an individual patient; and nurse and pharmacist independent prescribers to prescribe unlicensed medicines for their patients, on the same basis as doctors and dentists (and supplementary prescribers if part of a Clinical Management Plan).

**31** **Supplementary prescribing is a *voluntary* prescribing partnership between an *independent* prescriber and a *supplementary* prescriber.**

They do this to implement an agreed patient-specific Clinical Management Plan with patient agreement. The independent prescriber must be a doctor (or dentist).

**32** **The Medicines and Healthcare Products *Regulatory* Agency (MHRA) is a *government* agency.**

This agency is responsible for ensuring that medicines and medical devices work, and are acceptably safe. The MHRA is an executive agency of the Department of Health.

# 2 Drug development, marketing, and administration

## INTRODUCTION

Research and development of new drugs is paramount for enhancing both the health and wealth of the UK, and the pharmaceutical industry plays a key role in this. Patients in the National Health Service (NHS) have been major beneficiaries of the many therapeutic advances made by the pharmaceutical companies operating in the UK. Understanding the processes involved in the development and subsequent manufacture and supply of medicines is an important aspect of prescribing.

The overarching principles of safety, efficacy, and cost-effectiveness are paramount to a healthy population and economy, and as prescribers it is important to understand how these principles are put into practice. The process is complex, costly, and time-consuming, but a general understanding helps prescribers to be aware of the stringent regulations that govern and guide the process and ensures an understanding of the evidence base that underpins their prescribing. A sound knowledge of other factors that may have an impact on prescribing is also important if we are to prescribe safely and effectively.

### Useful resources

Association of the British Pharmaceutical Industry
www.abpi.org.uk

Medicines and Healthcare Products Regulatory Agency
www.mhra.gov.uk

## TRUE OR FALSE?

Are the following statements true or false?

**1** The packaging of a medication is governed by the same stringent controls as the active ingredient used in the drug.

**2** Phase I clinical trials are the first trials to be undertaken in humans.

**3** Medicines that meet the standards of safety, quality, and efficacy of the Medicine and Healthcare Products Regulatory Agency (MHRA) are granted a product licence.

**4** When drugs are added to infusion fluids for intravenous use, incompatibility is indicated by precipitation of the solutions.

**5** If an established medicine is to be used in a new patient population, the drug will be assigned Black Triangle (▼) status.

**6** Drug preparations that contain hydrogenated glucose syrup cannot be classed as 'sugar free'.

**7** The lactose content in a medicine should be ascertained before prescribing to patients with lactose intolerance.

**8** Advertising to the general public should not suggest that one product is better than another.

**9** POM, P, and GSL versions of the same generic product require different brand names.

**10** A prescriber can put a description of a medication (such as 'The Sleeping Tablets') on a prescription.

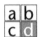

## MULTIPLE CHOICE

Identify one correct answer for each of the following.

**11** Codes of conduct and standards for promotional activities undertaken by pharmaceutical companies are set by:

a) the Medicine and Healthcare Products Regulatory Agency (MHRA)

b) the National Prescribing Centre (NPC)

c) the Association of the British Pharmaceutical Industry (ABPI)

d) the General Pharmaceutical Council (GPhC)

**12** The statement of ethical principles for medical research involving human subjects, including research on identifiable human material and data, is known as:

a) the Nuremberg Code

b) the Declaration of Helsinki

c) the Declaration of Geneva

d) the International Code of Medical Ethics

**13** The Declaration of Helsinki was drawn up by:

a) the World Medical Association (WMA)

b) the Medicine and Healthcare Products Regulatory Agency (MHRA)

c) the World Health Organization (WHO)

d) the International Code of Medical Ethics (ICME)

**14** Phase IV clinical trials are undertaken:

a) in healthy adults before a drug receives a licence

b) in healthy adults after a drug receives a licence

c) before a drug receives a licence and in patients with the disease to be treated by that drug

d) after a drug receives its licence and in patients with the disease to be treated by that drug

**15** The safety of all medicines is monitored throughout their marketed life by a process known as:

a) post-trials surveillance (PTS)

b) pharmacovigilance

c) pharmacopeia

d) post-marketing surveillance (PMS)

**16** Another name for the recommended international non-proprietary name (rINN) of a drug is:

a) adopted name

b) proprietary name

c) generic name

d) brand name

**17** For how long is a drug assigned Black Triangle (▼) status?

a) 2 years

b) 3 years

c) depends on the drug

d) depends on the evidence

**18** The Yellow Card Scheme is run by:

a) NPC and Department of Health

b) MHRA and Committee on Safety of Medicines (CSM)

c) Department of Health and CSM

d) MHRA and Commission on Human Medicines (CHM)

**19** The development of a drug in the UK costs approximately:

a) £350 million

b) £450 million

c) £550 million

d) £650 million

**20** An individual who both initiates and conducts a clinical trial is known as:

a) the investigator

b) the researcher

c) the coordinator

d) the monitor

**MATCH THE TERMS**

Match each term with the correct description.

- **A.** clinical trials authorization (CTA)
- **B.** protocol
- **C.** biotechnology
- **D.** List C
- **E.** posology
- **F.** extemporaneous preparation
- **G.** excipient

**21** Information on dosages of medicines and drugs.

**22** The document that describes the objective(s), design, methodology, statistical considerations, and organization of a trial.

**23** The industrial use of living organisms used in the production of drugs.

**24** Substances that are present in authorized products that have been reclassified since 1 April 2002.

**25** Consent by the MHRA and an ethics committee to allow clinical trials to take place.

**26** A mixture made to order (by prescription) rather than taken from stock.

**27** A pharmacologically inactive substance used as a carrier for the active ingredients of a medication.

## FILL IN THE BLANKS

Fill in the blanks in each statement using the options in the box.
*Not all of them are required, so choose carefully!*

| | |
|---|---|
| pre-packed | supply |
| specials | Council |
| crushing | the public |
| treating | summary |
| Medicines | plant |
| characteristics | preventing |
| supply | statutory |
| vegetable | |

**28** The _____ Act (1968) and _____ Directive 2001/83/EEC control the sale and _____ of medicines.

**29** SPC stands for _____ of product _____.

**30** General sale list (GSL) medicines are available from retail premises provided they are _____ and the premises concerned can be closed to exclude _____.

**31** The MHRA defines a medicine as 'any substance or combination of substances presented as having properties for _____ or _____ disease in human beings'.

**32** Herbal remedies are medicinal products consisting of a substance produced by subjecting a _____ or plants to drying, _____ or any other process.

**33** The law allows manufacture and _____ of unlicensed medicinal products (commonly known as '_____') subject to certain conditions.

# ANSWERS

## TRUE OR FALSE?

**1** | **The packaging of a medication is governed by the same stringent controls as the active ingredient used in the drug.**

The packaging of a medication is considered by the MHRA and forms part of the marketing authorization. Once a medication is removed from its packaging there is a breach of the terms of the licence, as the packaging has been altered.

**2** | **Phase I clinical trials are the first trials to be undertaken in humans.**

Trials are often undertaken in animals or on cells initially. The trials in humans then undergo a series of phases, Phase I being the initial phase that essentially looks at safety data and dosing. These trials are usually carried out on healthy volunteers/patients.

**3** | **Medicines that meet the standards of safety, quality, and efficacy of the Medicine and Healthcare Products Regulatory Agency (MHRA) are granted a product licence.**

This is now known as a marketing authorization.

**4** | **When drugs are added to infusion fluids for intravenous use, incompatibility is indicated by precipitation of the solutions.**

This may occur but in many cases there is no visual indication of incompatibility. Interaction may take place at any point and the potential for incompatibility is increased when more than one substance is added to the infusion fluid.

**5** | **If an established medicine is to be used in a new patient population, the drug will be assigned Black Triangle (▼) status.**

A product containing previously licensed active substances may also be monitored and assigned Black Triangle status: if it contains a new combination of active substances; if administration of the drug is via a new route of administration or a drug delivery system is required; if it is to be used for a significant new indication that may alter the established risk/benefit profile of that drug; or if it is an established medicine that is to be used in a new patient population.

**6** **Drug preparations that contain hydrogenated glucose syrup cannot be classed as 'sugar free'.**

Preparations containing hydrogenated glucose syrup, mannitol, maltitol, sorbitol or xylitol can be marked 'sugar free', since there is evidence that they do not cause dental caries.

**7** **The lactose content in a medicine should be ascertained before prescribing to patients with lactose intolerance.**

The British National Formulary (BNF) states that the lactose content in most medicines is too small to cause problems in the majority of lactose-intolerant patients. However, for sufferers of severe lactose intolerance and where medication is required, the manufacturers should be contacted to ascertain the specific lactose content of the medication to be prescribed and the recommendations regarding its use for such patients.

**8** **Advertising to the general public should not suggest that one product is better than another.**

The MHRA 'Blue Guide' (2005) states that advertising to the general public should not suggest that one product is better than (or equivalent to) another identifiable treatment or product, or that the effects of taking it are guaranteed. Material that refers in improper, alarming or misleading terms to claims of recovery must also not be included.

**9** **POM, P, and GSL versions of the same generic product require different brand names.**

As a result of changes brought about by the Medicines for Human Use and Medical Devices Regulations (2002), it is no longer possible to have more than one legal classification on a single marketing authorization. One effect of this is that POM, P, and GSL versions of the same product require different brand names. Where a change in legal classification is due only to a difference in pack size of the medicinal product but all other aspects of the marketing authorizations are the same, the same brand name can be used for the products.

**10** **A prescriber can put a description of a medication (such as 'The Sleeping Tablets') on a prescription.**

The BNF states that if a prescriber wishes to put a description of a tablet on the label of the medication, he or she can do so. This should not be used in place of the name of the medication but may be useful for patients to differentiate between their medication packaging.

# MULTIPLE CHOICE

Correct answers identified in bold italics.

**11** **Codes of conduct and standards for promotional activities undertaken by pharmaceutical companies are set by:**

a) the Medicine and Healthcare Products Regulatory Agency (MHRA)

b) the National Prescribing Centre (NPC)

*c) the Association of the British Pharmaceutical Industry (ABPI)*

d) the General Pharmaceutical Council (GPhC)

**12** **The statement of ethical principles for medical research involving human subjects, including research on identifiable human material and data, is known as:**

a) the Nuremberg Code

*b) the Declaration of Helsinki*

c) the Declaration of Geneva

d) the International Code of Medical Ethics

The Declaration of Helsinki was built on the Nuremberg Code after German physicians conducted medical experiments on thousands of concentration camp prisoners without their consent. The Declaration governs international research ethics and defines rules for 'research combined with clinical care' and 'non-therapeutic research'. It was last amended in 2008.

**13** **The Declaration of Helsinki was drawn up by:**

*a) the World Medical Association (WMA)*

b) the Medicine and Healthcare Products Regulatory Agency (MHRA)

c) the World Health Organization (WHO)

d) the International Code of Medical Ethics (ICME)

The World Medical Association was created to ensure the independence of physicians, and to work for the highest possible standards of ethical behaviour and care by physicians, at all times. The Declaration of Helsinki was adopted by the WMA General Assembly in 1964.

**14** **Phase IV clinical trials are undertaken:**

a) in healthy adults before a drug receives a licence

b) in healthy adults after a drug receives a licence

c) before a drug receives a licence and in patients with the disease to be treated by that drug

*d) after a drug receives its licence and in patients with the disease to be treated by that drug*

At this stage, the drugs are already on the market and being used, their safety having been established and having received a marketing authorization. Phase IV clinical trials are sometimes carried out to answer questions specific to one particular market, or to enable physicians to gain experience of a new drug under controlled conditions. They tend to be carried out in very large numbers of subjects and can be vital to establish a large comparative safety database for a drug. The most widely used type of Phase IV study is post-marketing surveillance (PMS), which is undertaken using the Yellow Card system of reporting.

**15** **The safety of all medicines is monitored throughout their marketed life by a process known as:**

a) post-trials surveillance (PTS)
b) *pharmacovigilance*
c) pharmacopeia
d) post-marketing surveillance (PMS)

Despite extensive research in animals and clinical trials in humans for a specific medicine, some adverse reactions may not be seen until a very large number of people have received the medicine. It is thus vital that the safety of all medicines is monitored continuously throughout the lifetime of their use; this monitoring is known as pharmacovigilance.

**16** **Another name for the recommended international non-proprietary name (rINN) of a drug is:**

a) adopted name   b) proprietary name
c) *generic name*   d) brand name

Each drug has an approved generic name. They will also have a proprietary or brand name, which is the name that the manufacturer uses for their specific brand of the generic drug. All drugs should be prescribed using the generic (or approved) name where possible, as this helps to reduce the incidence of error and can often be a more economical way of prescribing.

**17** **For how long is a drug assigned Black Triangle (▼) status?**

a) 2 years   b) 3 years   c) depends on the drug
d) *depends on the evidence*

The MHRA assesses the Black Triangle status of a product usually two years after marketing. However, there is no standard time for a product to retain Black Triangle status. The symbol is not removed until the safety of the drug is well established.

**18** **The Yellow Card Scheme is run by:**

a) NPC and Department of Health
b) MHRA and Committee on Safety of Medicines (CSM)

c)   Department of Health and CSM
**d)   MHRA and Commission on Human Medicines (CHM)**

The MHRA and the Commission on Human Medicines run the UK's spontaneous adverse drug reaction (ADR) reporting scheme, called the Yellow Card Scheme. This receives reports of suspected adverse drug reactions or side-effects from healthcare professionals and patients for medicines and vaccines. All Black Triangle drugs should have suspected ADRs reported using the Yellow Card Scheme.

**19**  **The development of a drug in the UK costs approximately:**

a)   £350 million   b) £450 million   *c) £550 million*   d) £650 million

The development of a drug in the UK takes approximately twelve years from start to finish, and costs approximately £550 million.

**20**  **An individual who both initiates and conducts a clinical trial is known as:**

*a)   the investigator*   b) the researcher   c) the coordinator
d)   the monitor

 **MATCH THE TERMS**

**21**  Information on dosages of medicines and drugs.   E. posology

**22**  The document that describes the objective(s), design, methodology, statistical considerations, and organization of a trial.   B. protocol

**23**  The industrial use of living organisms used in the production of drugs.   C. biotechnology

**24**  Substances that are present in authorized products that have been reclassified since 1 April 2002.   D. List C

**25**  Consent by the MHRA and an ethics committee to allow clinical trials to take place.   A. clinical trials authorization (CTA)

ANSWERS  *Drug development, marketing, and administration*

**26** A mixture made to order (by prescription) rather than taken from stock.

**F.** extemporaneous preparation

**27** A pharmacologically inactive substance used as a carrier for the active ingredients of a medication.

**G.** excipient

## FILL IN THE BLANKS

**28** The *Medicines* Act (1968) and *Council* Directive 2001/83/EEC control the sale and *supply* of medicines.

The legal status of medicinal products is part of the marketing authorization (MA) and products may be available on a prescription, in a pharmacy or on general sale.

**29** SPC stands for *summary* of product *characteristics*.

This is the data sheet provided with each drug by the manufacturer, which also corresponds to the information contained within the marketing authorization that a manufacturer submits to the MHRA. It is the definitive description of the drug both in terms of its properties and its indication.

**30** General sale list (GSL) medicines are available from retail premises provided they are *pre-packed* and the premises concerned can be closed to exclude *the public*.

Under the Medicines Act 1968, safety is the criterion for deciding the availability of a medicine. To protect public health, most medicines can only be sold or supplied at pharmacy premises by or under the supervision of a pharmacist. However, GSL medicines can be sold as long as they meet the criteria above. The term 'premises' is not defined but its ordinary meaning is a building or buildings with adjoining land.

**31** The MHRA defines a medicine as 'any substance or combination of substances presented as having properties for *treating* or *preventing* disease in human beings'.

They also add that any substance or combination of substances that may be used in or administered to human beings with a view to restoring, correcting or modifying physiological functions by exerting a pharmacological, immunological or metabolic action, or making a medical diagnosis is classed as a medicine.

**32** **Herbal remedies are medicinal products consisting of a substance produced by subjecting a _plant_ or plants to drying, _crushing_ or any other process.**

Section 13(2) of the Act defines a herbal remedy as 'a medicinal product consisting of a substance produced by subjecting a plant or plants to drying, crushing or any other process, or of a mixture whose sole ingredients are two or more substances so produced, or of a mixture whose sole ingredients are one or more substances so produced and water or some other inert substance'.

**33** **The law allows manufacture and _supply_ of unlicensed medicinal products (commonly known as '_specials_') subject to certain conditions.**

Some patients may have special clinical needs that cannot be met by licensed medicinal products. The conditions are that there is a bona fide unsolicited order, the product is formulated in accordance with the requirement of a doctor or dentist registered in the UK, and the product is for use by their individual patients on their direct personal responsibility.

# 3 Drug licensing and handling

## INTRODUCTION

Medicines have been regulated in various forms since the time of Henry VIII but it was not until 1971 that a comprehensive regulatory system was put in place (MHRA 2011). The Medicines Act 1968 collated and introduced new legal provision for medicines' safety and control. Linked to changes governing the legal and ethical principles of medical research, a system of licensing was developed that affected the manufacture, sale, supply, and importation of medicinal products into the UK, and it became unlawful to engage in these activities except in accordance with appropriate licences, certificates or exemptions. The Act was used specifically to provide a new system of licensing. Over time, European Union (EU) legislation has taken precedence over the Medicines Act (although there are regulations in the Act that are specific to the UK) and it is now the responsibility of the Medicines and Healthcare Products Regulatory Authority (MHRA) and the expert advisory bodies set up by the Medicines Act to ensure that drugs are safe and effective while also adhering to EU regulations.

Before a drug can be prescribed in the UK, it must be licensed and this process is undertaken by the MHRA, which assesses the safety, quality, and efficacy of the drug before granting a licence. Licensing issues are important for us as prescribers, as there are legal and ethical concerns that underpin our prescribing. This is never more apparent than when we are faced with the challenge of prescribing for groups of patients where the drugs we need are either unlicensed or not licensed for the particular indication, patient group or dose regime we need. Understanding the role of licensing in prescribing is vital if we are to ensure our own safe, effective, and evidence-based practice.

### Useful resources

Medicines and Healthcare Products Regulatory Agency
www.mhra.gov.uk

UK Medicines Information
www.ukmi.nhs.uk

European Medicines Agency
www.ema.europa.eu

**TRUE OR FALSE?**

Are the following statements true or false?

**1**    Crushing a tablet or opening a capsule prior to administration means the prescriber is using the drug off-licence.

**2**    All oral tablets and capsules can be put into a dosette box with no chance of drug deterioration.

**3**    Mixing two licensed medicines together in a syringe driver results in the prescriber prescribing an unlicensed medication.

**4**    Medicines added to a dosette box are still covered by the manufacturer's product licence.

**5**    Prescriptions for controlled drugs must be hand-written by the prescribing practitioner.

**6**    A drug fridge should contain a maximum/minimum thermometer and have readings recorded twice daily.

**7**    Most drugs used in neonatal medicine are used off-licence.

**8**    Premises where drugs are sold as general sales list medicines require a wholesale dealer's licence from the MHRA.

**9** Certain food products may be prescribed as long as they have ACBS (Advisory Committee on Borderline Substances) approval and are prescribed for the approved clinical condition outlined by the ACBS.

**10** To use amitriptyline for migraine prophylaxis, the prescriber would have to prescribe it off-licence.

**MULTIPLE CHOICE**

Identify one correct answer for each of the following.

**11** If a pharmaceutical company wishes to apply for a UK drug licence, they would apply to:

a) the European Medicines Agency (EMA)

b) the Medicines and Healthcare Products Regulatory Authority (MHRA)

c) the National Prescribing Centre (NPC)

d) the Committee on the Safety of Medicines (CSM)

**12** Unlicensed medications cannot be prescribed:

a) by a supplementary prescriber

b) by a nurse independent prescriber.

c) on a Patient Group Direction (PGD)

d) by a pharmacist independent prescriber

**13** The use of controlled drugs in medicine is permitted by:

a) the Misuse of Drugs Regulations 2001

b) the Misuse of Drugs Act 1971

c) the Committee on the Safety of Medicines

d) the Medicines Act 1968

**14** Dental nurses:

a) are allowed to prescribe for patients if the dentist authorizes it via a Clinical Management Plan (CMP)

b) are allowed to prescribe for patients if the dentist authorizes it via a PGD

   c)  are not allowed to prescribe in any circumstance

   d)  are allowed to prescribe dressings and simple pain analgesia

**15** Controlled drugs that can be prescribed by nurse independent prescribers include:

   a)  oral diazepam for muscle spasm

   b)  sublingual buprenorphine

   c)  oral morphine hydrochloride for pain relief in suspected myocardial infarction

   d)  all controlled drugs listed in Schedules 2–5

**16** Under the Medicines Act, which of the following is exempt from licensing?

   a)  off-licence medications

   b)  borderline substances

   c)  herbal remedies

   d)  excipients

**17** Master Jones is a 12-year-old boy with asthma. You decide to prescribe zafirlukast 20 mg twice daily for prophylaxis. In prescribing this drug for this child, you are prescribing:

   a)  off-licence

   b)  unlicensed

   c)  within its licence

   d)  off-label

**18** What is the approximate percentage of drugs in the UK that have not been licensed for use in children?

   a)  20%

   b)  30%

   c)  40%

   d)  50%

**19** A licence to manufacture unlicensed medicinal products and import unlicensed medicinal products from outside the European Economic Area is covered by:

a) a manufacturer's licence

b) a manufacturer's (specials) licence

c) a manufacturer's/importer's licence

d) a marketing authorization

**20** A Class I drug alert means that action should be taken:

a) immediately

b) within 24 hours

c) within 48 hours

d) within 5 days

**MATCH THE TERMS**

Match each term with the correct description.

    **A.** marketing authorization

    **B.** off-label drug

    **C.** manufacturer's licence

    **D.** complementary therapy

    **E.** parenteral

    **F.** schedule

    **G.** class

| **21** | Medicine with a product licence being used outside the terms of the licence. |

| **22** | Used to list drugs according to their harmfulness when misused. |

| **23** | A licence granted for medicines that meet the standards of safety, quality, and efficacy. |

| **24** | A licence granted following inspection of the manufacturing plant to ensure appropriate facilities and processes. |

| **25** | An additional substance, treatment or procedure used to increase the efficacy or safety of the primary substance, treatment or procedure, or to facilitate its performance. |

| **26** | Not via the digestive system. |

| **27** | Used to define who is authorized to supply and possess controlled drugs. |

## FILL IN THE BLANKS

Fill in the blanks in each statement using the options in the box.
*Not all of them are required, so choose carefully!*

| | |
|---|---|
| routes | safeguard |
| devices | pharmacologically |
| developed | acceptable |
| named | indications |
| borderline | acceptably |
| rare | pharmaceutical |
| equivalent | approved |

**28** MHRA's mission is to enhance and _____ the health of the public by ensuring that medicines and medical _____work, and are _____ safe.

**29** For a food supplement to be classed as a _____ product, it must contain a _____ active substance.

**30** An orphan drug is a _____ agent that is _____specifically to prevent or treat a _____ medical condition.

**31** Unlicensed prescribing is _____ so long as it is considered best practice and where no _____ alternative is available, and is generally used on a _____ patient basis.

# ANSWERS

## TRUE OR FALSE?

**1** | **Crushing a tablet or opening a capsule prior to administration means the prescriber is using the drug off-licence.**

Tampering with a medicine before administration (for example, by crushing or dispersal) will render it to be off-licence (see p. 37) if not recommended by the manufacturer in the data sheet. In such circumstances, the responsibility for any adverse effects the patient may suffer rests largely with the prescriber. It is therefore important that any decision to recommend off-licence medicine use is considered best practice, with informed patient consent and appropriate documentation.

**2** | **All oral tablets and capsules can be put into a dosette box with no chance of drug deterioration.**

Once a medication is removed from its packaging, deterioration begins almost immediately, particularly if tablets are removed from blister packs.

**3** | **Mixing two licensed medicines together in a syringe driver results in the prescriber prescribing an unlicensed medication.**

All licensed medicines have been tested for effectiveness and safety before being released onto the market. The data sheet provided by the pharmaceutical company with any licensed medication states the conditions whereby the drug has been proven to be safe in the patient group if given at the recommended dose and via the recommended route in the form in which it was tested. If these conditions are altered in any way, the prescriber will be working without a licence – for example, the addition of a second active drug means the two effectively become one new drug without a licence.

**4** | **Medicines added to a dosette box are still covered by the manufacturer's product licence.**

When drugs are taken out of their packaging and placed into a dosette box, there is a breach of the terms of the manufacturer's licence as the packaging has changed.

**5** | **Prescriptions for controlled drugs must be hand-written by the prescribing practitioner.** ✖

It is now acceptable for controlled drug prescriptions to be computer-generated or written by other personnel. However, it is best practice for them to be written or generated by a suitably qualified health professional and they *must* be signed by the prescribing practitioner.

**6** | **A drug fridge should contain a maximum/minimum thermometer and have readings recorded twice daily.**

The minimum requirement for temperature monitoring is for a thermometer that measures maximum and minimum temperatures to be placed within the load, so that as far as possible it is not affected by repeatedly opening and closing the door. The thermometer should be read and reset daily and the maximum and minimum temperatures recorded.

**7** | **Most drugs used in neonatal medicine are used off-licence.**

Because clinical trials with infants and children are viewed as unethical, most medications are licensed in the UK but do not have a licence for use in these age groups and therefore are used off-licence.

**8** | **Premises where drugs are sold as general sales list medicines require a wholesale dealer's licence from the MHRA.**

Companies that are involved in all stages of the manufacture and distribution of a drug need to have a licence (manufacturer's licence and wholesale dealer's licence). Applications for a manufacturer's and wholesale dealer's licence require an inspection by the MHRA Inspectorate to ensure the premises and procedures are up to the requisite quality standards.

**9** | **Certain food products may be prescribed as long as they have ACBS (Advisory Committee on Borderline Substances) approval and are prescribed for the approved clinical condition outlined by the ACBS.**

Certain foods (and toilet preparations) have characteristics of drugs and the ACBS advises as to the circumstances in which these substances may be regarded and therefore prescribed as drugs. Prescriptions for these substance must be endorsed 'ACBS'.

**10** | **To use amitriptyline for migraine prophylaxis, the prescriber would have to prescribe it off-licence.**

Amitriptyline has a marketing authorization for depressive illness, although the British National Formulary (BNF) states it is not recommended for use for this indication. Amitriptyline is most often used for neuropathic pain and migraine prophylaxis, although it does not have a licence for these indications and is therefore used off-licence. *Note*: The BNF states 'unlicensed' against these indications; however, unlicensed and 'off-label' (off-licence) medicines are all shown with the term 'unlicensed'. Therefore, good knowledge of the terms unlicensed and off-licence is important for the prescriber to be able to make an informed decision.

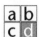 **MULTIPLE CHOICE**

Correct answers identified in bold italics.

**11** If a pharmaceutical company wishes to apply for a UK drug licence, they would apply to:

a) the European Medicines Agency (EMA)

*b) the Medicines and Healthcare Products Regulatory Authority (MHRA)*

c) the National Prescribing Centre (NPC)

d) the Committee on the Safety of Medicines (CSM)

**12** Unlicensed medications cannot be prescribed:

a) by a supplementary prescriber

b) by a nurse independent prescriber

*c) on a Patient Group Direction (PGD)*

d) by a pharmacist independent prescriber

Since 2005, supplementary prescribers have been able to prescribe unlicensed medications as long as they form part of a Clinical Management Plan. Nurse and pharmacist independent prescribers have been able to prescribe unlicensed medications since the changes in legislation implemented in 2009.

**13** The use of controlled drugs in medicine is permitted by:

*a) the Misuse of Drugs Regulations 2001*

b) the Misuse of Drugs Act 1971

c) the Committee on the Safety of Medicines

d) the Medicines Act 1968

The drugs are classified in five schedules according to different levels of control. The Misuse of Drugs Act 1971 imposes total prohibition on the import and export, manufacture, supply, and possession of these drugs.

**14** Dental nurses:

a) are allowed to prescribe for patients if the dentist authorizes it via a Clinical Management Plan (CMP)

b) are allowed to prescribe for patients if the dentist authorizes it via a PGD

*c) are not allowed to prescribe in any circumstance*

d) are allowed to prescribe dressings and simple pain analgesia

**15** **Controlled drugs that can be prescribed by nurse independent prescribers include:**

a)  oral diazepam for muscle spasm

b)  sublingual buprenorphine

c)  oral morphine hydrochloride for pain relief in suspected myocardial infarction

d)  *all controlled drugs listed in Schedules 2–5*

Changes to the Misuse of Drugs Regulations 2001 relating to nurse and pharmacist independent prescribing of controlled drugs (*Misuse of Drugs (Amendment No. 2) (England, Wales and Scotland) Regulations 2012 (Statutory Instrument 2012/973)*), which came into force on 23 April 2012, enable nurse independent prescribers to prescribe any controlled drug listed in Schedules 2–5 for any medical condition within their competence. The exceptions are diamorphine, cocaine, and dipipanone for the treatment of addiction (nurse independent prescribers are able to prescribe other controlled drugs for the treatment of addiction). Nurse independent prescribers are able to requisition controlled drugs and are authorized to possess, supply, offer to supply, and administer the drugs they are able to prescribe. Persons acting in accordance with the directions of a nurse independent prescriber are authorized to administer any Schedules 2–5 drugs that the nurse can prescribe.

**16** **Under the Medicines Act, which of the following is exempt from licensing?**

a)  off-licence medications    b)  borderline substances

c)  *herbal remedies*    d)  excipients

The Medicines Act contains certain important exemptions from licensing and makes provision for further exemptions to be included in statutory orders. These exemptions also include: the manufacture and supply of unlicensed relevant medicinal products for individual patients ('specials'); the importation and supply of unlicensed relevant medicinal products for individual patients; and herbal remedies.

**17** **Master Jones is a 12-year-old boy with asthma. You decide to prescribe zafirlukast 20 mg twice daily for prophylaxis. In prescribing this drug for this child, you are prescribing:**

a)  off-licence   b)  unlicensed   c)  *within its licence*   d)  off-label

This drug is licensed for use with adults and children over 12 years, and thus would be within the licence for this indication and at this dose. *Note*: 'Off-label' is another term for 'off-licence'.

**18** **What is the approximate percentage of drugs in the UK that have not been licensed for use in children?**

a)   20%   b) 30%   c) 40%   *d) 50%*

The MHRA suggests that over 50% of the medicines used in children may not have been studied in this age group. In the European Union, the paediatric population (0–18 years) represents about 75 million people, which is 20% of the total population.

**19** **A licence to manufacture unlicensed medicinal products and import unlicensed medicinal products from outside the European Economic Area is covered by:**

a)   a manufacturer's licence
*b)   a manufacturer's (specials) licence*
c)   a manufacturer's/importer's licence
d)   a marketing authorization

If a 'special' is manufactured in the UK, the manufacturer must hold a manufacturer's (specials) licence issued by the MHRA. A 'special' may not be advertised and may not be supplied if an equivalent licensed product is available that meets the patient's needs. Essential records must be kept and serious adverse drug reactions reported to the MHRA.

**20** **A Class I drug alert means that action should be taken:**

*a)   immediately*   b)   within 24 hours
c)   within 48 hours   d)   within 5 days

Where a defective medicine is considered to present a risk to public health, the marketing authorization holder or the manufacturer as appropriate, is responsible for recalling the affected batch(es) or, in extreme cases, removing all batches of the product from the market. These alerts are issued by the MHRA's Defective Medicines Report Centre (DMRC).

# MATCH THE TERMS

**21**   Medicine with a product licence being used outside the terms of the licence.

B.   off-label drug

**22**   Used to list drugs according to their harmfulness when misused.

G.   class

**23** A licence granted for medicines that meet the standards of safety, quality, and efficacy.

**A.** marketing authorization

**24** A licence granted following inspection of the manufacturing plant to ensure appropriate facilities and processes.

**C.** manufacturer's licence

**25** An additional substance, treatment or procedure used to increase the efficacy or safety of the primary substance, treatment or procedure, or to facilitate its performance.

**D.** complementary therapy

**26** Not via the digestive system.

**E.** parenteral

**27** Used to define who is authorized to supply and possess controlled drugs

**F.** schedule

## FILL IN THE BLANKS

**28** **MHRA's mission is to enhance and _safeguard_ the health of the public by ensuring that medicines and medical _devices_ work, and are _acceptably_ safe.**

**29** **For a food supplement to be classed as a _borderline_ product, it must contain a _pharmacologically_ active substance.**

A product that is for use only as a toilet preparation, disinfectant, food or beverage is not normally regarded as a medicinal product, and therefore does not require a marketing authorization according to the MHRA before being sold in the UK. Similarly, dietary supplements containing substances such as vitamins, amino acids or minerals are generally subject to food safety and food labelling legislation rather than medicines control.

**30** An orphan drug is a *pharmaceutical* agent that is *developed* specifically to prevent or treat a *rare* medical condition.

The condition itself is referred to as an orphan disease. In the USA and European Union, it is easier to gain marketing approval for an orphan drug, and often medical breakthroughs have occurred that may not have done had the costly research and development process been undertaken in the usual process of drug development.

**31** Unlicensed prescribing is *acceptable* so long as it is considered best practice and where no *equivalent* alternative is available, and is generally used on a *named* patient basis.

Under the current legislation, a healthcare professional can decide to treat a patient with a medicine that is not licensed where there is a special clinical need. Special clinical need means that there is no equivalent medication or formulation of that medication available, or where a previously held licence has been relinquished or where a drug is likely to be unavailable for a significant period. Prescribers must take full responsibility for their actions and have gained informed consent from the patient.

# 4 Getting to know your BNF

## INTRODUCTION

When starting prescriber training, most students are familiar with the British National Formulary (BNF). It is an ever-present book in the work environment and is used regularly, if not necessarily the latest edition. Despite some familiarity with the BNF, most students are unaware of the information that it contains. It is used as a reference to ascertain a drug dose or the price of one drug compared with an alternative.

The BNF is much more than a list of drugs and the doses that should be used for a particular condition. It contains a wealth of information about the licensed drugs in the UK, as well as guidance on their use, drug interactions, and general prescribing advice. The aim of this chapter is to make the reader more aware of the information that is contained within this important resource. The answers to the questions are all contained within the BNF. Thus it is expected that at the end of this chapter, the reader will be more aware and have a better understanding of the information that is contained within its pages. The BNF is also available online at www.bnf.org.

> **Useful resources**
>
> British National Formulary
> www.bnf.org

**TRUE OR FALSE?**

Are the following statements true of false?

**1** Borderline substances are foods or nutritional supplements that are considered drugs when they are used for the management of specified conditions.

**2** Older adults are more sensitive to the action of drugs on the nervous system, such as opioid analgesics, benzodiazepines, and antipsychotics.

**3** When prescribing in palliative care, parenteral administration of a drug by continuous infusion is indicated when the patient does not wish to take medication by mouth.

**4** In the BNF, the recommended international non-proprietary name (rINN) is always the same as the British Approved Name (BAN).

**5** Information about cautionary and advisory labels can be found in Appendix 9.

**6** You can prescribe Mrs Crimbles' gluten-free cheesecake mix on an FP10.

**7** You are allowed to mix ondansetron with diamorphine in a syringe driver.

**8** Buprenorphine can be prescribed sublingually by a non-medical prescriber for palliative care.

**9** There is an increased risk of ventricular arrhythmias when tricyclic anti-depressants are given with amiodarone.

**MULTIPLE CHOICE**

Identify one or more correct answer from each of the following.

**10** Which of the following is *not* recommended when writing a prescription?

a) quantities less than 1 gram should be written in milligrams

b) preparations to be taken 'as required' should specify a minimum dose interval

c) computer-generated signatures meet legal requirements

d) never abbreviate the units

**11** Which of the following is *not* recommended in the BNF as a measure to prevent adverse reactions?

a) avoid prescribing if the patient is already taking over-the-counter or herbal medicine

b) prescribe as few drugs as possible

c) with a new drug, be alert for adverse drug reactions or unexpected events

d) alert the patient if adverse reactions are liable to occur

**12** The BNF suggests that creatinine clearance can be calculated using:

a) the Duckworth-Lewis formula

b) the Cockcroft-Gault formula

c) the Henderson-Hasselbalch formula

d) the Galton and Simpson formula

**13** What should a non-medical prescriber do if he or she suspects a case of drug misuse in the UK?

a) notify the National Drug Treatment Monitoring System (NDTMS)

b) notify the Substance Misuse Programme (SMP)

  c) notify the Chief Medical Officer (CMO)

  d) notify the National Database for Substance Misuse (NDSM)

**14** Which of the following drugs does the BNF say can be mixed with diamorphine?

a) hyoscine hydrochloride

b) hydrocortisone

c) levopromazine

d) temazepam

**15** Which of the following are potential interactions with iron preparations?

a) reduced excretion of oral iron with antacids

b) reduced absorption of oxytetracycline with oral iron preparations

c) reduced metabolism of aspirin with oral iron

d) reduced absorption of iron with calcium channel blockers

**16** Which are the recommended instructions for the labels of a prescription for soluble paracetamol tablets?

a) do not take anything containing aspirin while taking this medicine

b) dissolve or mix with water before taking

c) do not take with any other paracetamol products

d) do not take more than 2 at any one time. Do not take more than 8 in 24 hours

**17** What is the name of the organization that provides information and advice on poisons?

a) Poisons Control Centre

b) Medicines and Healthcare Products Regulatory Agency

c) Drug Safety Agency

d) National Poisons Information Service

**18** What type of substance is P K Aid 4?

   a)  fluid and electrolyte replacement used for diabetic ketoacidosis

   b)  borderline substance used for phenylketonuria

   c)  substance used to reduce absorption of poisons from the gastro-intestinal tract

   d)  non-proprietary name for a stimulant laxative


**19** How many Yellow Card Centres are there that can be contacted for further information about an adverse reaction to a drug?

   a)  3

   b)  4

   c)  5

   d)  6


**20** Information on the use of intramuscular adrenaline for anaphylaxis can be found in:

   a)  Section 3.4.1

   b)  Section 3.4.2

   c)  Section 3.4.3

   d)  all of the above


**21** The Nurse Prescribers' Formulary is a list of preparations approved by:

   a)  the Secretary of State

   b)  the Medicines and Healthcare Products Regulatory Authority (M H R A)

   c)  the Royal Pharmaceutical Society

   d)  the Nursing and Midwifery Council (N M C)

**22** Which route can morphine hydrochloride be prescribed by a non-medical prescriber?

a) orally

b) rectally

c) parenterally

d) all of the above

**23** What change in dose needs to be made to Cefaclor for a patient with renal impairment?

a) no change, manufacturer advises caution

b) half the normal dose

c) if estimated glomerular filtration rate is less than 5 mL/min/1.73 m$^2$, halve normal dose

d) start with half normal dose and increase to full dose after 24 hours

**24** What problems should be monitored when using syringe drivers?

a) rate of infusion

b) battery

c) injection site reaction

d) all of the above

**25** What can aminophylline be added to for intravenous infusion?

a) water

b) 5% glucose solution

c) 0.9% NaCl

d) 5% glucose solution and 0.9% NaCl

**26** What does cautionary label number 1 state?

 a) do not drink alcohol

 b) dissolve or mix with water before taking

 c) this medicine may make you sleepy

 d) do not drive or use tools or machines

**LABELLING EXERCISE**

Label the symbols or abbreviations below:

27

28 ▼

29 POM

30 ●

31

# FILL IN THE BLANKS

Fill in the blanks in each statement using the options in the box.
*Not all of them are required, so choose carefully!*

| | |
|---|---|
| acetylcysteine | cautionary |
| 50 | regulatory |
| charcoal | 72 |
| short-term | proper |
| blood | bone marrow |
| 32 | 100 |
| thrombotic | poisons |
| 96 | methionine |

**32** The maximum number of paracetamol tablets a nurse can prescribe is _____ tablets with a maximum pack size of _____ tablets.

**33** When prescribing for older adults, drug-induced _____ disorders are more common and may cause _____ _____ depression.

**34** The _____ officer should be informed if you suspect a patient of having a notifiable disease.

**35** The two drugs used for treatment of paracetamol overdose are _____ and _____.

**36** The maximum number of aspirin (antiplatelet) tablets that can be sold to the public is _____ tablets.

**37** When prescribing non-selective NSAIDs, the cautionary advice is that there is a 'small increase in the risk of _____ episodes' even with _____ use.

# ANSWERS

## TRUE OR FALSE?

**1** Borderline substances are foods or nutritional supplements that can be considered drugs when they are used for the management of specified conditions.

Borderline substances in Appendix 2 of the BNF can be regarded as drugs and may be prescribed for the management of specified conditions, provided that the prescriber is satisfied that they are safe and that the patient is adequately monitored.

**2** Older adults are more sensitive to the action of drugs on the nervous system, such as opioid analgesics, benzodiazepines, and antipsychotics.

This is true and the drugs should therefore be used with caution as stated in the section on prescribing for older adults in the BNF. It is also true for other groups of drugs, such as the antihypertensives on the cardiovascular system. This is due to the effect of ageing on pharmacokinetics, which reduces the clearance of drugs from the body.

**3** When prescribing in palliative care, parenteral administration of a drug by continuous infusion is indicated when the patient does not wish to take medication by mouth.

The section in the BNF on prescribing in palliative care provides advice on the use of continuous infusion devices. There are three indications for using this particular route of administration: (1) the patient is unable to take medicines by mouth because of nausea and vomiting, dysphagia, weakness or coma; (2) there is a malignant bowel obstruction; (c) the patient does not wish to take regular medication by mouth.

**4** In the BNF, the recommended international non-proprietary name (rINN) is always the same as the British Approved Name (BAN).

The rINN for medicinal substances is the name that is required to be used by European law. The BAN and the rIIN are often the same. However, changes to the names of some medicines have been made to reduce the risk of a prescribing or dispensing error. Examples of changes to names include: lignocaine to lidocaine, frusemide to furosemide, and oestradiol to estradiol. There are two exceptions to this rule: adrenaline and noradrenaline are the terms used in the European Pharmacopoeia but the rINNs are epinephrine and norepinephrine, respectively. A full list of the names of substances affected by this change can be found at:

http://www.mhra.gov.uk/Howweregulate/Medicines/Namingofmedicines/ChangestomedicinesnamesBANstorINNs/index.htm.

**5** **Information about cautionary and advisory labels can be found in Appendix 9.**

The information on cautionary labels is found in Appendix 3.

**6** **You can prescribe Mrs Crimbles' gluten-free cheesecake mix on an FP10.**

The BNF does contain Mrs Crimbles' gluten-free products but not a cheesecake mix.

**7** **You are allowed to mix ondansetron with diamorphine in a syringe driver.**

Under the section on prescribing in palliative care, there is a list of drugs that can be mixed with diamorphine. However, ondansetron is not one of them.

**8** **Buprenorphine can be prescribed sublingually by a non-medical prescriber for palliative care.**

Buprenorphine can only be prescribed transdermally for palliative care.

**9** **There is an increased risk of ventricular arrhythmias when tricyclic antidepressants are given with amiodarone.**

Appendix 1 of the BNF contains a list of drug interactions. It advises that concomitant use of amiodarone and tricyclic antidepressants should be avoided.

 **MULTIPLE CHOICE**

Correct answers identified in bold italics

**10** **Which of the following is *not* recommended when writing a prescription?**

a) quantities less than 1 gram should be written in milligrams
b) preparations to be taken 'as required' should specify a minimum dose interval
c) *computer-generated signatures meet legal requirements*
d) never abbreviate the units

| 11 | **Which of the following is *not* recommended in the BNF as a measure to prevent adverse reactions?** |

a) *avoid prescribing if the patient is already taking over-the-counter or herbal medicine*

b) prescribe as few drugs as possible

c) with a new drug, be alert for adverse drug reactions or unexpected events

d) alert the patient if adverse reactions are liable to occur

There is a section in the BNF that provides information on adverse drug reactions and measures to prevent their occurrence. It suggests asking patients if they take over-the-counter or herbal preparations and to use a few drugs as possible, but does not suggest avoiding prescribing.

| 12 | **The BNF suggests that creatinine clearance can be calculated using:** |

a) the Duckworth-Lewis formula

*b) the Cockcroft-Gault formula*

c) the Henderson-Hasselbalch

d) the Galton and Simpson formula formula

The section on prescribing in renal impairment gives the Cockcroft-Gault formula for estimating creatinine clearance.

| 13 | **What should a non-medical prescriber do if he or she suspects a case of drug misuse in the UK?** |

a) *notify the National Drug Treatment Monitoring System (NDTMS)*

b) *notify the Substance Misuse Programme (SMP)*

c) *notify the Chief Medical Officer (CMO)*

d) *notify the National Database for Substance Misuse (NDSM)*

The answer is dependent on where in the UK the practitioner is located. In England, prescribers should report drug misuse to the National Drug Treatment Monitoring System team; in Scotland, to the Substance Misuse Programme. In Northern Ireland, the information should be sent to the Chief Medical Officer of the Department of Health and Social Services. In Wales, the information should be sent to the Welsh National Database for Substance Misuse. These are similar reporting systems. Their addresses are contained in the section at the front of the BNF on Controlled Drugs and Drug Dependence.

| 14 | **Which of the following drugs does the BNF say can be mixed with diamorphine?** |

a) hyoscine hydrochloride   b) hydrocortisone

c) *levopromazine*   d) temazepam

At the end of the section on Prescribing in Palliative Care, there is a table that indicates which drugs can be mixed with diamorphine.

**15**   **Which of the following are potential interactions with iron preparations?**

a) reduced excretion of oral iron with antacids

b) *reduced absorption of oxytetracycline with oral iron preparations*

c) reduced metabolism of aspirin with oral iron

d) reduced absorption of iron with calcium channel blockers.

Appendix 1 of the BNF contains a long list of interactions between two or more drugs. Interactions can also be found in the online BNF. Additional information regarding individual drugs can be found immediately under the drug's name. This provides a link to the interactions for the named drug.

Interactions can be pharmacodynamic in nature – that is, the drugs have a similar mode of action or have an antagonistic effect.

Other interactions are pharmacokinetic in nature, affecting the absorption, distribution, metabolism or excretion of another drug. These interactions can increase or decrease the effectiveness of the drug or the duration of action the drug has in the body. Many drug interactions are relatively harmless but others can be serious. Therefore, it is good practice to look up the potential interactions of drugs newly added to a medication regimen and to anticipate potential problems.

**16**   **Which are the recommended instructions for the labels of a prescription for soluble paracetamol tablets?**

a) do not take anything containing aspirin while taking this medicine

b) *dissolve or mix with water before taking*

c) *do not take with any other paracetamol products*

d) *do not take more than 2 at any one time. Do not take more than 8 in 24 hours*

Appendix 3 of the BNF contains the codes for the cautionary and advisory labels for dispensed medicines. These are the labels recommended for use by the pharmacist when dispensing medicines. The appendix contains a list of the products and the codes for the labels as well as advice about administration of the drug. Soluble paracetamol tablets are a paediatric dispersible formulation containing 120 mg of drug. The advisory label code is 13, 29, 30. The wording can be found in Appendix 3 and also inside the back pages. So the dispensed medicines label should contain the words from options (b), (c), and (d).

**17**   **What is the name of the organization that provides information and advice on poisons?**

a) Poisons Control Centre

b) Medicines and Healthcare Products Regulatory Agency

c) Drug Safety Agency

*d) National Poisons Information Service*

The UK National Poisons Information Service is the organization that should be consulted if advice is needed about the risk and management of poisonings. The BNF provides basic information on the emergency treatment of poisoning in a chapter before the sections on Drugs and Preparations. The chapter has basic advice on how to handle the episode and information on the products that can be used for some cases of poisoning. The service has developed a database of clinical toxicological knowledge called TOXBASE that is available to registered users via the Internet.

**18** **What type of substance is PK Aid 4?**

a) fluid and electrolyte replacement used for diabetic ketoacidosis

*b) borderline substance used for phenylketonuria*

c) substance used to reduce absorption of poisons from the gastro-intestinal tract

d) non-proprietary name for a stimulant laxative

Appendix 2 contains a comprehensive list of substances considered as borderline substances that have the characteristics of drugs in certain circumstances.

**19** **How many Yellow Card Centres are there that can be contacted for further information about an adverse reaction to a drug?**

a) 3   b) 4   *c) 5*   d) 6

There are five centres in the UK that can be contacted for further information: Liverpool, Cardiff, Newcastle upon Tyne, Edinburgh, and Birmingham. See the section on Adverse Reactions to Drugs.

**20** **Information on the use of intramuscular adrenaline for anaphylaxis can be found in:**

a) Section 3.4.1   b) Section 3.4.2   *c) Section 3.4.3*   d) all of the above

**21** **The Nurse Prescribers' Formulary is a list of preparations approved by:**

*a) the Secretary of State*

b) the Medicines and Healthcare Products Regulatory Authority (MHRA)

c) the Royal Pharmaceutical Society

d) the Nursing and Midwifery Council (NMC)

After the appendices in the BNF, there is a section on the Nurse Prescribers' Formulary.

**22** | **Which route can morphine hydrochloride be prescribed by a non-medical prescriber?**

*a) orally*   b)   rectally   c)   parenterally   d)   all of the above

Morphine is available as several salts in the BNF. Morphine hydrochloride is only available as an oral preparation.

**23** | **What change in dose needs to be made to Cefaclor for a patient with renal impairment?**

*a)  no change, manufacturer advises caution*

b)   half the normal dose

c)   if estimated glomerular filtration rate is less than 5 mL/min/1.73 m$^2$, halve normal dose

d)   start with half normal dose and increase to full dose after 24 hours

**24** | **What problems should be monitored when using syringe drivers?**

a) rate of infusion    b)   battery   c)   injection site reaction

*d) all of the above*

The section on Prescribing in Palliative Care provides advice on the problems that can be encountered with syringe drivers.

**25** | **What can aminophylline be added to for intravenous infusion?**

a) water   b)   5% glucose solution   c)   0.9% NaCl

*d) 5% glucose solution and 0.9% NaCl*

Appendix 4 provides a table of drugs given by intravenous infusion and details how the drugs should be prepared.

**26** | **What does cautionary label number 1 state?**

a) do not drink alcohol

b) dissolve or mix with water before taking

*c)  this medicine may make you sleepy*

d) do not drive or use tools or machines

Cautionary labels are detailed in Appendix 3 and the wording in brief is found inside the back page.

**LABELLING EXERCISE**

**27**

This symbol is used to indicate when the Joint Formulary Committee considers the preparation 'to be less suitable for prescribing'. The preparation may not be the best one to use as a drug of first choice.

**28**

The black triangle symbol identifies a preparation that is being 'monitored intensively by the M H R A'.

**29** POM

The P O M symbol indicates that these preparations are only available on a prescription issued by an appropriately trained practitioner.

**30** ●

Potentially serious drug interaction, this combination of drugs should be avoided.

**31**

A preparation that is in Schedule 3 of the Misuse of Drugs Regulations 2001 (and subsequent amendments).

## FILL IN THE BLANKS

**32** | The maximum number of paracetamol tablets a nurse can prescribe is _96_ tablets with a maximum pack size of _32_ tablets.

The Nurse Prescribers' Formulary section in the BNF has a footnote that indicates the maximum number of paracetamol tablets that can be prescribed is 96 in packs of 32. However, pharmacists can sell to the public multiple packs of 32 up to a total quantity of 100 tablets or capsules; see footnote in Section 4.7.1.

**33** | When prescribing for older adults, drug-induced _blood_ disorders are more common and may cause _bone marrow_ depression.

In the Guidance on Prescribing chapter in the BNF, there is a section on prescribing for older adults, which lists some of the adverse reactions often found in this group of patients.

**34** | The _proper_ officer should be informed if you suspect a patient of having a notifiable disease.

At the start of Section 5 on Infections, advice is provided on whom the practitioner should inform when a patient is suspected of a notifiable disease.

**35** | The two drugs used for treatment of paracetamol overdose are _methionine_ and _acetylcysteine_.

The chapter in the BNF on Emergency Treatment of Poisoning gives detailed information on how to treat an overdose of paracetamol as well as other drugs. This section also provides links to TOXBASE and the National Poisons Information Service.

**36** | The maximum number of aspirin (antiplatelet) tablets that can be sold to the public is _100_ tablets.

To be found in the footer of Section 2.9; up to a hundred 75 mg tablets may be sold to the public.

**37** | When prescribing non-selective NSAIDs, the cautionary advice is that there is a 'small increase in the risk of _thrombotic_ episodes' even with _short-term_ use.

In Section 10.1.1 under Cautions and Contra-indications, there is a highlighted box on NSAIDs and cardiovascular events, which provides advice on the use of cyclo-oxygenase-2 selective and non-selective NSAIDs and the associated cardiovascular risk.

# 5 Legal and ethical issues in prescribing

## INTRODUCTION

Ethics provides a framework within which difficult issues can be resolved in a moral way. There may be several outcomes and paths down which a practitioner can proceed. The law, which provides the rules by which society is expected to live, is constantly modified as society identifies issues that are not adequately addressed by or fall outside of existing legislation.

Ethics and the law do not always complement each other. The law can be changed and moral beliefs may also change as society changes. Modern scientific and medical developments raise a wealth of issues as novel situations arise. Without some guidance or an ethical framework, the best interests of individuals and society cannot be met.

The increased use of medicines in society has raised many new ethical dilemmas, particularly in relation to the cost of and access to these medicines. The prescriber may need to consider what the law will allow and what may be in the best interests of the patient. This chapter provides questions that test the prescriber's understanding of the ethical and legal aspects of non-medical prescribing.

> **Useful resources**
>
> Medicines and prescribing support from NICE
> www.nice.org.uk/mpc/index.jsp
>
> Nursing and Midwifery Council (NMC)
> www.nmc-uk.org

**TRUE OR FALSE?**

Are the following statements true of false?

**1** A prescription is a legal document.

**2** Under the Mental Capacity Act 2005, a non-medical prescriber cannot assume a patient has capacity to agree to treatment until proven.

**3** If a prescriber advises a patient to obtain an over-the-counter medication, the prescriber is not accountable for any problem that may occur.

**4** Prescribers are accountable for not giving adequate advice about prescribed medicines.

**5** Patients who are unable to swallow pills can have their medicines crushed to help them take their medication.

**6** Non-medical prescribers can only prescribe unlicensed medications under a Clinical Management Plan.

**7** The law does not allow non-medical prescribers to prescribe unlicensed drugs to children.

**8** The Bolam test is applied to judge if a treatment is considered 'best practice'.

**9** The Bolitho test is used in British legal cases to determine if medical negligence has occurred.

**10** A non-medical prescriber cannot issue an emergency prescription for a controlled drug.

**11** A nurse independent prescriber can prescribe and give instructions to mix diamorphine with cyclizine in a syringe driver.

**12** A person is deemed to lack capacity to consent if they are unable to make a decision.

**13** The Gillick Guidelines relate specifically to contraception in the under-16s.

**14** Consent is an ongoing process that does not need reaffirming.

**MULTIPLE CHOICE**

Identify one correct answer from each of the following.

**15** In which year was the law changed to allow community nurses to prescribe?

a) 1992

b) 1998

c) 2005

d) 2006

**16** Which of the following Acts of Parliament allows non-medical prescribers to prescribe from all of the British National Formulary?

a) Medicinal Products: Prescription by Nurses and Others Act 1992

b) Prescription Only Medicines Order (Human Use) 1997

c) Medicines and Human Use (Prescribing) (Miscellaneous Amendments) Order 2006

d) the Medicines for Human Use (Miscellaneous Amendments) (No. 2) Regulations 2009

**17** Which of the following are required for a legal prescription of a POM under the Medicines Act 1968?

a) signature of prescriber (in ink), full name of patient, full address of patient, address of prescriber, date

b) signature of prescriber (in ink), full name of patient, address of prescriber, date, age of patient

c) signature of prescriber (in ink), full address of patient, date, age of patient, total quantity supplied

d) signature of prescriber (in ink), address of prescriber, date, total quantity prescribed, strength of medicine

**18**　Which of the following can an independent non-medical prescriber prescribe for the treatment of addictions?

a) diamorphine

b) dipipanone

c) cocaine

d) diazepam

**19**　Under the Mental Capacity Act 2005, a person may lack capacity for a number of reasons. Which of the following options is *not* a reason to deem an adult lacks capacity?

a) concussion after a head injury

b) deafness

c) learning disabilities

d) symptoms of drug or alcohol use

**20**　Which of the following activities does the Misuse of Drugs Act 1971 prohibit in relation to controlled drugs?

a) manufacture

b) possession

c) supply

d) all of the above

**21**　When prescribing a controlled drug, how long is the prescription valid for?

a) 48 hours

b) 21 days

c) 28 days

d) 30 days

**MATCH THE TERMS**

Match each term with the correct description:

    **A.** beneficence
    **B.** autonomy
    **C.** deontology
    **D.** fidelity
    **E.** justice
    **F.** non-maleficence
    **G.** accountability
    **H.** veracity
    **I.** utilitarianism

**22** Liability for one's own actions.

**23** Moral obligation regardless of consequences for human welfare.

**24** Obligation to keep promises.

**25** Responsibility to tell the truth.

**26** Requirement to do good.

**27** Obligation to avoid harm.

**28**  Duty to be fair and equitable in the entitlement to care.

**29**  Principle of the greatest good for the greatest number of people.

**30**  The right of individuals to make choices for themselves.

# FILL IN THE BLANKS

Fill in the blanks in each statement using the options in the box.
*Not all of them are required, so choose carefully!*

| | |
|---|---|
| unlicensed | prescription-only |
| duty of care | competent |
| adequately | obligation |
| controlled | contraception |
| illegal | capacity |
| confidentiality | consent |
| voluntarily | |

**31** All _____ drugs are _____ medicines under the Medicines Act 1968.

**32** The Fraser Guidelines relate specifically to _____ in the under-16 age group.

**33** Informed _____ is an ongoing agreement to receive treatment after the risks and benefits have been _____ explained to a patient.

**34** Practitioners are under a legal and ethical _____ to maintain _____ of information given in confidence.

**35** The practitioner who is prescribing for a patient owes that patient a _____ .

**36** Consent is an agreement given _____ by a mentally _____ person.

# ANSWERS

## TRUE OR FALSE?

**1** **A prescription is a legal document.**

Under the provisions of the Medicines Act 1968, a prescription is a legal document.

**2** **Under the Mental Capacity Act, a non-medical prescriber cannot assume a patient has capacity to agree to treatment until proven.**

The practitioner must assume that the patient has capacity unless it is established that they lack the capacity.

**3** **If a prescriber advises a patient to obtain an over-the-counter medication, the prescriber is not accountable for any problem that may occur.**

The practitioner is accountable for both actions and omissions. As a qualified prescriber, the practitioner is accountable for the advice he or she gives to take any medicine, whether prescribed or over-the-counter.

**4** **Prescribers are accountable for not giving adequate advice about prescribed medicines.**

As the practitioner is accountable for both actions and omissions, he or she is accountable for not giving adequate advice about medications.

**5** **Patients who are unable to swallow pills can have their medicines crushed to help them take their medication.**

Although this may occur in practice, the medicines having been crushed become an unlicensed medicine, as they are not in the approved formulation. The prescriber would not usually prescribe crushed medication and so the medicine is not as directed.

**6** **Non-medical prescribers can only prescribe unlicensed medications under a Clinical Management Plan.**

Following amendments to the Medicines for Human Use Act in December 2009, independent non-medical prescribers are allowed to prescribe unlicensed medicines. However, optometrist prescribers are not able to prescribe unlicensed medicines.

**7** | **The law does not allow non-medical prescribers to prescribe unlicensed drugs to children.**

Like the previous answer, independent non-medical prescribers are able to prescribe unlicensed medicines. Many drugs are unlicensed for children but may be licensed for adults because clinical trials have not been completed on children for ethical reasons.

**8** | **The Bolam test is applied to judge if a treatment is considered 'best practice'.**

The Bolam test is applied to test if there has been a breach in the duty of care to a patient. It compares the care given with accepted standards of care given by an equivalently trained professional.

**9** | **The Bolitho test is used in British legal cases to determine if medical negligence has occurred.**

The Bolitho test has superseded the Bolam test in medical negligence cases. It requires that evidence supports professional opinions and that the evidence is judged to be reasonable, respectable or responsible.

**10** | **A non-medical prescriber cannot issue an emergency prescription for a controlled drug.**

It is allowable to prescribe controlled drugs in an emergency only for extreme pain.

**11** | **A nurse independent prescriber can prescribe and give instructions to mix diamorphine with cyclizine in a syringe driver.**

The Misuse of Drugs (Amendment No. 2) Regulations 2012 made changes allowing independent non-medical prescribers to prescribe, administer, and give directions for the administration of Schedules 2, 3, 4, and 5 controlled drugs for the treatment of organic disease or injury.

**12** | **A person is deemed to lack capacity to consent if they are unable to make a decision.**

Under the Mental Capacity Act 2005, a person lacks capacity if they are unable to make a decision because of impairment or disturbance in the functioning of their brain. This may be a temporary or permanent disturbance.

**13** | **The Gillick Guidelines relate specifically to contraception in the under-16s.**

*Gillick* v. *West Norfolk and Wisbech Area Health Authority* 1985 established a principle that under-16s, if deemed 'Gillick competent', have the right to seek confidential medical advice and make their own decisions without their parents' knowledge or consent. While the case was about doctors giving contraceptive advice, Gillick competence has wider implications for confidentiality and the autonomy of competent under-16s. As a result of a High Court appeal, Lord Fraser provided guidelines that apply specifically to contraceptive advice and treatment to under-16s.

**14 Consent is an ongoing process that does not need reaffirming.**

Consent is an agreement given by a mentally competent person, voluntarily without coercion. It needs reaffirming whenever a decision or treatment is to be given. A patient may have given consent previously, but may change their mind later. The patient has the right to be autonomous even if their decision conflicts with clinical practice.

# MULTIPLE CHOICE

Correct answers identified in bold italics.

**15 In which year was the law changed to allow community nurses to prescribe?**

*a) 1992*   b)   1998   c)   2005   d)   2006

The Medicinal Products: Prescription by Nurses and Others Act 1992 allowed prescribing by health visitors and district nurses. This gave access to a limited range of drugs and was amended in 1994 with a revised list of medicines published in the Nurse Prescribers' Formulary.

**16 Which of the following Acts of Parliament allows non-medical prescribers to prescribe from all of the British National Formulary?**

a)   Medicinal Products: Prescription by Nurses and Others Act 1992

b)   Prescription Only Medicines Order (Human Use) 1997

*c)   Medicines and Human Use (Prescribing) (Miscellaneous Amendments) Order 2006*

d)   the Medicines for Human Use (Miscellaneous Amendments) (No. 2) Regulations 2009

The 1992 Act allowed prescribing by health visitors and district nurses. The 1997 Order introduced supplementary prescribing. In 2006, the Miscellaneous Amendments Order removed some limitations to nurse and pharmacist prescribers and allowed them to prescribe from all of the BNF, provided it was within their scope of experience. The changes in 2009 allowed independent non-medical prescribers to mix medicines and prescribe unlicensed medicines (but not controlled drugs).

**17** **Which of the following are required for a legal prescription of a POM under the Medicines Act 1968?**

a) *signature of prescriber (in ink), full name of patient, full address of patient, address of prescriber, date*

b) signature of prescriber (in ink), full name of patient, address of prescriber, date, age of patient

c) signature of prescriber (in ink), full address of patient, date, age of patient, total quantity supplied

d) signature of prescriber (in ink), address of prescriber, date, total quantity prescribed, strength of medicine

The Medicines Act requires relatively few details for a prescription to be valid. The age and date of birth of a patient are only required if they are under 12 years. However, it is usual practice to include the date of birth of the patient.

**18** **Which of the following can an independent non-medical prescriber prescribe for the treatment of addictions?**

a) diamorphine  b)  dipipanone  c)  cocaine  **d)  *diazepam***

Amendments to the Misuse of Drugs Regulations came into force in April 2012 and allowed nurse and pharmacist independent prescribers to prescribe Schedule 2, 3, 4, and 5 controlled drugs, provided that they are within their scope of practice. However, the amendments did not include the prescribing of diamorphine, dipipanone or cocaine for the treatment of addictions, which is restricted to Home Office licensed doctors.

**19** **Under the Mental Capacity Act 2005, a person may lack capacity for a number of reasons. Which of the following options is *not* a reason to deem an adult lacks capacity?**

a) concussion after a head injury   **b) *deafness***

c) learning disabilities   d) symptoms of drug or alcohol use

While deafness can be a permanent disability, it does not impair the person's cognitive ability to make a decision, whereas the other conditions can impair a person's ability to make rational decisions. It is up to the practitioner to judge whether the person's cognitive function is impaired.

**20** **Which of the following activities does the Misuse of Drugs Act 1971 prohibit in relation to controlled drugs?**

a) manufacture  b)  possession  c)  supply  **d)  *all of the above***

The Act defines the types of persons who, while acting in their professional capacity and under what circumstances, are able to possess and supply controlled drugs.

**21** **When prescribing a controlled drug, how long is the prescription valid for?**

a) 48 hours   b) 21 days   *c) 28 days*   d) 30 days

A prescription for any controlled drug (excluding those in Schedule 5) is valid for 28 days.

 **MATCH THE TERMS**

**22** Liability for one's own actions.

**G.** accountability

**23** Moral obligation regardless of consequences for human welfare.

**C.** deontology

**24** Obligation to keep promises.

**D.** fidelity

**25** Responsibility to tell the truth.

**H.** veracity

**26** Requirement to do good.

**A.** beneficence

**27** Obligation to avoid harm.

**F.** non-maleficence

**28** Duty to be fair and equitable in the entitlement to care.

**E.** justice

**29** Principle of the greatest good for the greatest number of people.

**I.** utilitarianism

**30** The right of individuals to make choices for themselves.

**B.** autonomy

# FILL IN THE BLANKS

**31** All _controlled_ drugs are _prescription-only_ medicines under the Medicines Act 1968.

The Medicines Act 1968 sets out the three categories of medicines (general sales; pharmacy; prescription-only medicines) under this scheme; all controlled drugs are considered prescription-only medicines. However, there are exemptions to the Act that allow some health professionals to supply and administer some controlled drugs.

**32** The Fraser Guidelines relate specifically to _contraception_ in the under-16 age group.

These guidelines are useful in determining the strategy of contraceptive treatment of a person under 16 years. They also need to be deemed 'Gillick or Fraser competent' for them to make their own treatment choices.

**33** Informed _consent_ is an ongoing agreement to receive treatment after the risks and benefits have been _adequately_ explained to a patient.

For consent to be valid, the person must have the capacity to make a decision, be fully informed of the risks and benefits of a treatment, and the consent must be given voluntarily. As consent is a continuous process, the person has the right to change their mind regarding treatment. So once consent is given, it is not irreversible.

**34** Practitioners are under a legal and ethical _obligation_ to maintain _confidentiality_ of information given in confidence.

This principle is universal in healthcare. The Department of Health publication *Confidentiality: NHS Code of Practice* (2003) sets out the duty of healthcare professionals within the organization. Without confidentiality, the patient may lose trust.

**35** The practitioner who is prescribing for a patient owes that patient a _duty of care_.

It is a legal principle that healthcare professionals owe their patients a duty of care and should act in accordance with accepted practice. If they breach that duty of care, they may be deemed negligent.

**36** Consent is an agreement give _voluntarily_ by a mentally _competent_ person.

If a person is not mentally competent, they will lack the capacity to give consent. For consent to be valid, it must also be given voluntarily without 'deceit or fraud'.

# 6 Principles of pharmacology

## INTRODUCTION

Pharmacology is the science behind prescribing. It is 'the study of the actions and effects of drugs on physiological systems' (Galbraith et al., 2007). It is important for prescribers to have an understanding of the principles of pharmacology in order to use drugs effectively in the clinical setting. As a prescriber, you need to know which mechanisms are affected by a drug in its therapeutic action on the body, as well as understanding what the body does to the drug on its journey through the body.

The actions drugs have on the body are known as *pharmacodynamics*, while the processes undertaken by the body on the drug are termed *pharmacokinetics*. Students are often put off by complicated words. As with many subjects, once they can see through the language and understand the principles of pharmacology, it become easier. One of our students had a 'light-bulb moment' and declared, 'I get it now – pharmacology is physiology with drugs!' While the subject is more complicated than this, a good knowledge of the biological sciences will help you to understand how drugs interact with the different systems of the body to produce their effects. The aim of this chapter is to test understanding of the principles of drug actions.

### Useful resources

Barber, P. and Robertson, D. (2012) *Essentials of Pharmacology for Nurses*, 2nd edn. Maidenhead: Open University Press.

Galbraith, A., Bullock, S., Manias, E., Hunt, B. and Richards, A. (2007) *Fundamentals of Pharmacology: An Applied Approach for Nursing and Health*, 2nd edn. Harlow: Prentice-Hall.

*Nurses! Test Yourself in Pharmacology*

## TRUE OR FALSE?

Are the following statements true or false?

**1** An agonist binds reversibly to a competitive antagonist to block its action.

**2** A receptor binds reversibly with naturally occurring neurotransmitters and hormones.

**3** A receptor transports molecules across membranes.

**4** Lipid solubility is an important factor affecting the rate of absorption of a drug.

**5** Absorption of a drug is unaffected by the acidity of the gastrointestinal tract.

**6** A receptor converts chemical signals into cellular responses.

**7** Drugs such as aspirin inhibit enzymes.

**8** Drugs that block reuptake systems can enhance the action of neurotransmitters.

**9** The first pass effect refers to the proportion of drug absorbed in passing through the stomach to the intestine.

**10** Drug metabolites can be active and inactive pharmacologically.

**11** Phase II of drug metabolism involves conjugation with metabolites.

**12** Genetics can affect the way drugs are metabolized by the body.

**13** Kidney disease can increase drug clearance from the body.

**14** Plasma protein binding delays the excretion of a drug.

**15** Age has no effect on the distribution of drugs.

**16** Drugs with a narrow therapeutic index have a small range of doses to give optimum clinical effects.

**MULTIPLE CHOICE**

Identify one correct answer for each of the following.

**17** An agonist can:

a) block a hormone

b) inhibit an enzyme

c) cause a biological response

d) block an ion channel

**18** Antagonists block the response to:

a) an agonist

b) an enzyme

c) calcium channels

d) transport systems

**19** The half-life of a drug is defined as:

a) half the time a drug is used in a course of treatment

b) half the time between drug doses

c) the time taken for the concentration of a drug to fall by 50%

d) the time taken for the concentration of a drug to increase by 50%

**20** A drug is said to be selective if:

a) it binds to one set of receptors

b) it binds to one cell type

c) it binds to receptors but doesn't activate them

d) it binds to one type of receptors at small concentrations

**21** Which of the following is *not* a phase of pharmacokinetics?

a) absorption

b) distribution

c) metabolism

d) exclusion

**22** Phase I of drug metabolism involves:

a) polarization

b) myoglobin

c) cytochromes

d) hydrophobes

**23** A pro-drug is:

a) an active metabolite

b) an inducer of metabolism

c) a long-acting formulation

d) an antidote

**24** Excretion of drugs by the kidney

a) declines with age

b) increases with age

c) is unaffected by age

d) is fully functional at birth

**25** Drug metabolism of a patient can be affected by:

a) pH of blood

b) drug half-life

c) nutritional status

d) competitive antagonism

**26** The volume of distribution is a measure of:

a) the apparent volume of the intracellular space

b) the volume of the plasma

c) the apparent volume within which a drug is dissolved in the body

d) the apparent volume of the lipid compartment in the body

**MATCH THE TERMS**

Match each term with the correct description:

A. absorption
B. pharmacokinetics
C. metabolism
D. agonists
E. bioavailability
F. pharmacodynamics
G. antagonists
H. plasma proteins

**27** What a drug does to the body.

**28** The effects of the body on drugs.

**29** Naturally occurring chemicals in the body.

**30** Chemicals that block responses to neurotransmitters.

**31** The proportion of drug available in the bloodstream.

**32** These reduce the free concentration of drugs in the circulation.

**33** Chemical alteration of drugs in the body.

**34** Passage of drug from the site of administration to the bloodstream.

**FILL IN THE BLANKS**

Fill in the blanks in each statement using the options in the box.
*Not all of them are required, so choose carefully!*

| | | |
|---|---|---|
| absorption | less potent | higher |
| membranes | liver | antagonist |
| decreasing | excretion | lower |
| full agonist | inhibit | metabolites |
| partial agonist | more potent | agonist |
| increasing | kidney | pharmacokinetics |

Use Figure 6.1 to answer Questions 35–37.

**Figure 6.1 Dose–response graph**

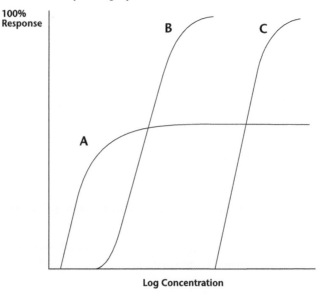

**35** Drug A is a ____ ____ .

**36** Drug B is a ____ ____ .

**37** Drug C is ____ ____ than drug B.

**38** An agonist can overcome the effects of an antagonist by _____ the concentration of the agonist.

**39** Morphine is an _____ and naloxone is an _____ of opiate receptors.

**40** Cyclizine is an _____ of histamine, used to treat nausea and vomiting.

**41** A potent drug requires a _____ concentration to bind to a receptor.

**42** In general, fat-soluble drugs cross cell _____ quicker than water-soluble drugs.

**43** The _____ is the principal site of drug metabolism.

**44** Some drugs that _____ drug metabolism can prolong the duration of action of drugs.

**45** Older adults and neonates have different _____ to young adults.

# ANSWERS

## TRUE OR FALSE?

**1** **An agonist binds reversibly to a competitive antagonist to block its action.**

Competitive antagonism involves the interaction of the agonist and the antagonist with a receptor. The agonist and antagonist both have affinity for the receptor and can therefore bind to it. The antagonist blocks the action of the agonist by interfering with the binding of the agonist with the receptor and 'gets in the way' of the agonist. The agonist can only elicit a response when it binds with the receptor; by interfering with the binding to the receptor, the antagonist lessens the agonist response. Drugs that bind together can reduce the effectiveness of each other by a chemical interaction. This is not competitive antagonism.

**2** **A receptor binds reversibly with naturally occurring neurotransmitters and hormones.**

The neurotransmitters and hormones are the natural agonists in the body. The process of binding of the receptor and an agonist is a dynamic phenomenon. The receptor has a binding site with a structure that is complementary to the chemical structure of the agonist and there is an innate attraction by the agonist for the receptor. The ability of the receptor and agonist to associate is often compared with a lock and a key mechanism. The dynamic nature of the agonist and receptor binding means that the process is reversible. The ease of binding of the agonist to the receptor is dependent on how 'sticky' they are (this is called the affinity of the agonist for the receptor). The probability of a receptor being activated by an agonist is dependent on the concentration of the agonist and the affinity the agonist has for the receptor.

**3** **A receptor transports molecules across membranes.**

Receptors are not molecular transport mechanisms. The action of an agonist on the receptor leads to changes on the inside of a cell membrane. The receptor is a transducer converting the binding of an agonist on the outside of the cell into a biological effect on the inside of the cell. Transport systems bind the substance being transported on one side of the cell membrane and by a change in the structure of the transporter it passes the substance to the other side of the membrane. This process may need energy to facilitate the transportation, e.g. proton pumping in the stomach.

**4** **Lipid solubility is an important factor affecting the rate of absorption of a drug.**

For drugs to be absorbed, they need to cross membranes in the body. The cell membrane is a lipid environment that excludes water and charged particles. Drugs that are soluble in lipids are 'lipophillic' (liking the lipid environment and hating water, or 'hydrophobic'). Drugs that are lipid soluble are not charged or ionized and like the environment within the cell membrane and can easily pass into the cell membrane. They can pass from one side of the cell down a concentration gradient from a high concentration on one side to a lower concentration on the other, using the lipid environment of the cell membrane. Lipid solubility is therefore an important factor in the absorption of drugs.

**5** **Absorption of a drug is unaffected by the acidity of the gastrointestinal tract.**

Drugs that are polar or are charged at physiological pH are influenced by the acidity or alkalinity of the environment in which they are found. Drugs that are acidic will be charged at physiological pH (7.4). In an acid environment, the drug will lose its charge and become uncharged or non-polar. In this state, drugs can pass through the non-polar environment of the cell membrane. The pH of the environment from which a drug is absorbed can be an important factor in the rate of drug absorption.

**6** **A receptor converts chemical signals into cellular responses.**

A receptor is a transducer that converts the binding of an agonist on the outside of the cell into a biological effect on the inside of the cell. It detects the chemical signal on the outside of the cell and turns it into a signal on the inside of the cell that leads to the overall cellular response. This may be the contraction of muscle, the secretion of a gland or the change in the activity of a neurone.

**7** **Drugs such as aspirin inhibit enzymes.**

Aspirin is one of the non-steroidal anti-inflammatory drugs (NSAIDs) that inhibit the cyclooxygenase family of enzymes. This results in the reduction of prostaglandins that mediate inflammatory processes. It is an example of a drug that inhibits a particular type of target molecules. There are many other examples of drugs that are used clinically to inhibit enzymes. However, inhibiting these enzymes can also have predictable side effects that the prescriber must also be aware of and take into account when prescribing. The NSAIDs also reduce prostaglandins' production in the stomach that can lead to ulceration, and in the kidney can lead to salt and water retention.

**8** **Drugs that block reuptake systems can enhance the action of neurotransmitters.**

Some of the commonly used anti-depressives drugs are known to block the reuptake of the neurotransmitters serotonin (5-HT), noradrenaline, and dopamine in the central nervous system. These drugs block the transporter that recovers the neurotransmitter present in synapses in the brain and allows it to be recycled. Serotonin selective reuptake inhibitors (SSRIs) are perhaps the best known of this category of drugs. By inhibiting the reuptake, the concentration of the neurotransmitter in the synapse builds up and enhances the action of the neurotransmitter on its receptors in the synapse.

### 9 | The first pass effect refers to the proportion of drug absorbed in passing through the stomach to the intestine.

The first pasts effect refers to the metabolism of a drug in passing through the gut and the liver, before it reaches the systemic circulation. Only drugs that are given orally are really affected by this process and it is also referred to as pre-systemic elimination. The net result is that not all the drug that is administered reaches the systemic circulation; much of it gets metabolized before it can have an effect on its target. The classic example of a drug that is affected by first pass metabolism is glyceryl trinitrate (GTN). To avoid this effect, GTN needs to be given by a route that avoids the gut or the liver.

### 10 | Drug metabolites can be active and inactive pharmacologically.

The objective of Phase I metabolism is to change the structure of the parent drug molecule. This usually reduces the activity of the drug for its target. However, some metabolic conversions do not make the drug metabolite inactive, as the metabolites can have pharmacological activity themselves. This tends to prolong the duration of the drug in the body.

### 11 | Phase II of drug metabolism involves conjugation with metabolites.

Phase II drug metabolism takes the drug metabolite created during Phase I and combines it with another highly water-soluble molecule. This makes the metabolites at the end of Phase II much more water-soluble. The metabolite can now be easily filtered by the kidney and excreted in the urine.

### 12 | Genetics can affect the way drugs are metabolized by the body.

The genetic make-up of an individual has many effects, including the cytochrome p450 enzymes utilized in drug metabolism. There are several versions of the cytochrome p450 enzymes that a person can inherit. Some of these forms are better than others at metabolizing some drugs. The genetic make-up of a patient affects the way that he or she metabolizes certain drugs, which may account for differences in the way patients respond to drug therapy and why some individuals are more susceptible to side effects while others appear not to respond very well.

### 13 Kidney disease can increase drug clearance from the body.

Disease that affects the renal blood flow or mass of the kidney reduces the capacity of the kidney to filter blood plasma and influences the glomerular filtration rate (GFR). This will reduce the capacity of the body to clear the drug and its metabolites from the system.

### 14 Plasma protein binding delays the excretion of a drug.

Drugs can easily bind with the circulating plasma proteins. The binding of drugs and plasma protein does not produce any physiological response and thus these proteins are not a molecular target for drug action. The binding of a drug to plasma proteins can be as much as 99% of the total amount of the drug in the body, leaving very small amounts free to have a pharmacological effect. The binding of the drug to these proteins also means that the drug is held in the plasma and is not available to be metabolized or to be excreted. The drug will therefore remain in the body for a longer period of time and will have a longer half-life than if it was not bound to the plasma proteins.

### 15 Age has no effect on the distribution of drugs.

Children have a higher proportion of their body weight as water and as we grow older we increase the proportion of the body that is fat. Older adults also experience a decrease in muscle mass. This affects the way that water- and lipid-soluble drugs are distributed in the body. For instance, diazepam is a lipid-soluble drug that has a different distribution in an adult because there is a smaller proportion of body fat in children. In the very young and in older adults there are fewer plasma proteins, which reduces the plasma protein binding of drugs, increasing the proportion of drug that is free and available to have an action. In neonates, the blood–brain barrier is not fully formed, which allows hydrophilic drugs to act when they would not normally penetrate into the brain. Therefore age affects the distribution of drugs in the body.

### 16 Drugs with a narrow therapeutic index have a small range of doses to give optimum clinical effects.

The therapeutic index (TI) is used to determine the range of concentrations at which a drug can be used, between the therapeutically effective concentration and a concentration that produces unwanted effects. It is calculated by dividing the maximum non-toxic dose by the minimum effective dose:

$$TI = \text{maximum non-toxic dose/minimum effective dose.}$$

This gives an indication of how wide a range of doses can be used clinically before side effects are observed. A drug with a much higher maximum non-toxic dose compared with the minimum effective dose will have a higher TI and therefore will have a greater safety margin than a drug with a small TI. Drugs that have a small TI will need to be used carefully and they must be monitored to ensure that the toxic effects of the drug are minimized. Sometimes the range of doses is referred to as the therapeutic window.

# MULTIPLE CHOICE

Correct answers identified in bold italics.

**17** **An agonist can:**

a)   block a hormone   b)   inhibit an enzyme

c)   *cause a biological response*   d)   block an ion channel

Agonists can be naturally occurring hormones and neurotransmitters in the body as well as drugs. They bind to receptors on cells and activate them to cause a biological response.

**18** **Antagonists block the response to:**

*a)*   *an agonist*   b)   an enzyme   c)   calcium channels

d)   transport systems

An antagonist is also a drug that binds to receptors on cells, but unlike an agonist it does not activate the receptor. The binding of the antagonist interferes with the binding of an agonist to the receptor and is said to block the response of the agonist.

**19** **The half-life of a drug is defined as:**

a)   half the time a drug is used in a course of treatment

b)   half the time between drug doses

c)   *the time taken for the concentration of a drug to fall by 50%*

d)   the time taken for the concentration of a drug to increase by 50%

The rate of elimination of a drug is a combination of the metabolism and the excretion of the drug from the body. The half-life is a measure of a drug's elimination from the blood and usually has units of hours. The half-life is defined as the time taken for the initial concentration of the drug to fall by 50%. This measure is useful to know when determining how often a drug should be given to patients. Doses that are too close together will result in a build-up of drug in the body and could lead to the development of side effects of the drug. If doses are given too far apart, the concentration of the drug in the body can fall below the level considered to be effective therapeutically.

**20** **A drug is said to be selective if:**

a)   it binds to one set of receptors

b)   it binds to one cell type

c) it binds to receptors but doesn't activate them

**d) it binds to one type of receptors at small concentrations**

Many drugs can bind to a variety of receptor types and are said to have affinity for these receptors. The affinity for a receptor can be measured and quantified experimentally. A drug that is selective for one receptor type will bind to that receptor at very small concentrations. At higher concentrations the drug may also bind to several other receptor types. Thus a drug has the ability to bind to many receptors but a selective drug at therapeutic levels will only bind to the desired receptor to have its effect. However, if the drug is given at too high a dose, then a drug effect can be detected from other receptors. This could result in a side effect being seen. A non-selective drug can have effects on several receptors at therapeutic levels. For example, salbutamol is a selective $\beta_2$ adrenoreceptor agonist and will act on the receptors in the bronchiole but will have little or no effect on the $\beta_1$ adrenoreceptors in the heart. However, if too much salbutamol is taken or too many doses are taken, too close together, then it may stimulate $\beta_1$ receptors and increase the heart rate.

**21** **Which of the following is *not* a phase of pharmacokinetics?**

a) absorption   b) distribution   c) metabolism   **d) exclusion**

The four phases of pharmacokinetics are absorption, distribution, metabolism, and excretion.

**22** **Phase I of drug metabolism involves:**

a) polarization   b) myoglobin   **c) cytochromes**   d) hydrophobes

Drug metabolism occurs primarily in the liver and has two phases. Phase I consists of a process where the drugs are oxidized, reduced or broken in two (hydrolysis). There is a large family of enzymes that metabolize drugs and other chemicals absorbed by the body; these enzymes are known as the cytochrome P450 superfamily. The cytochromes are important co-factors in the catalytic process of these enzymes.

**23** **A pro-drug is:**

**a) an active metabolite**   b) an inducer of metabolism

c) a long-acting formulation   d) an antidote

A pro-drug is a chemical that, when given to a person, does not have biological activity. The drug undergoes metabolism and is changed chemically. This change to the molecule makes a metabolite that is biologically active. Some drugs are designed to be pro-drugs and some apparently active drugs have been discovered to be pro-drugs. The analgesic codeine is a pro-drug that is converted into its active metabolite morphine.

## 24 Excretion of drugs by the kidney

*a) declines with age*　b)　increases with age

c) is unaffected by age　d)　is fully functional at birth

Kidney function declines with age. A neonate's kidney function is substantially lower than that of an adult. During the first year of life, the kidney reaches its full functional ability and then declines gradually through life. The decline in function reduces the ability of the body to clear drugs from the system.

## 25 Drug metabolism of a patient can be affected by:

a) pH of blood　b)　drug half-life

*c) nutritional status*　d)　competitive antagonism

Drug metabolism is primarily affected by the enzyme function of the liver in Phase I (cytochrome P450 enzymes) and conjugation in Phase II of metabolism. Anything that affects these enzymes will change the way that drugs are metabolized by the body. Enzymes are pH sensitive but changes in the blood pH do not affect liver enzyme function. The nutritional status of a person can have a marked influence on metabolism. If a person is malnourished, they may lack vitamins in the diet. Vitamins are vital for the normal functions of the body. Many vitamins are important co-factors in the chemical conversion of drugs to inactive metabolites. Protein malnourishment will affect the amount and composition of the plasma proteins. Changes in the plasma proteins will affect the capacity of those proteins to bind drugs. Both of these effects will result in higher concentrations of drug in the body. The half-life of the drug is a measure of how long the drug remains in the body; it does not influence metabolism.

## 26 The volume of distribution is a measure of:

a)　the apparent volume of the intracellular space

b)　the volume of the plasma

*c)　the apparent volume within which a drug is dissolved in the body*

d)　the apparent volume of the lipid compartment in the body

Once absorbed into the systemic circulation, drugs are distributed into the tissues. Depending on the chemical nature of the drug, it can be contained in several compartments in the body, i.e. plasma, fat or specific tissues such as the brain. The volume that contains the drug in the body is called the volume of distribution ($V_d$), and is calculated from the known drug dose and by measuring the concentration of the drug in the plasma:

$$V_d = \text{amount of drug in the body/concentration of drug in the plasma}$$

This is a theoretical value and can be larger than the volume of the body. This volume can tell us if the drug is concentrated in one of the body compartments or whether it is contained mostly in the water phase of the plasma. Drugs with a small apparent volume of distribution are concentrated in the blood, whereas drugs with a large apparent volume of distribution are concentrated in another part of the body such as the fat component. This can have clinical consequences for the calculation of a loading dose of a drug or in the case of an overdose. Drugs that have a large volume of distribution have a long duration of action.

 **MATCH THE TERMS**

| 27 | What a drug does to the body. | F. | pharmacodynamics |

| 28 | The effects of the body on drugs. | B. | pharmacokinetics |

| 29 | Naturally occurring chemicals in the body. | D. | agonists |

| 30 | Chemicals that block responses to neurotransmitters. | G. | antagonists |

| 31 | The proportion of drug available in the bloodstream. | E. | bioavailability |

| 32 | These reduce the free concentration of drugs in the circulation. | H. | plasma proteins |

| 33 | Chemical alteration of drugs in the body. | C. | metabolism |

| 34 | Passage of drug from the site of administration to the bloodstream. | A. | absorption |

# FILL IN THE BLANKS

**Figure 6.1 Dose–response graph**

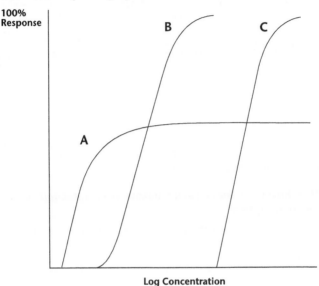

**Log Concentration**

| 35 | Drug A is a _partial agonist_. |

| 36 | Drug B is a _full agonist_. |

The dose–response graph in Figure 6.1 shows the relationship between the concentration of a drug and the percentage of the maximal response obtained from the tissue. Drugs A, B, and C all produce responses from the tissue and are therefore agonists. A drug that produces the maximal tissue response is called a full agonist. As can be seen on the graph, drugs B and C cause the maximum response, whereas drug A does not, even at the highest concentrations. Drug A is called a partial agonist, as it only produces a partial response from the tissue.

| 37 | Drug C is _less potent_ than drug B. |

The graph also shows that drug A can cause a tissue response at lower concentrations than either drug B or drug C. Drug A is therefore more potent than drug B because it binds to the receptors to cause a response at a lower concentration, and thus has a higher affinity for the receptor than drug B. Drug C does not cause a response until the concentration of the drug is much higher than the concentration that causes a response from drug B. Drug C is therefore less potent than drug B. Drug B therefore has a higher affinity for the receptors involved than drug C.

**38** **An agonist can overcome the effects of an antagonist by** *increasing* **the concentration of the agonist.**

Competitive antagonists have affinity for receptors. They have a chemical shape that allows them to bind to the same site on receptors that also bind an agonist. The way an agonist acts on a receptor is similar to that of a lock and a key, the receptor being the lock and the agonist the key. If the key has the right shape, it can fit into the lock and open it. The antagonist is like a badly cut key – it can fit into the lock but cannot open it, and when in the lock the bad key prevents a good key from opening the lock. The process in reality is much more dynamic than a single lock and a key because there are many locks and millions more keys involved. The keys are constantly trying to open the locks. The probability of a receptor being activated is dependent on the concentration of the agonist. If an antagonist is also present, it will also bind to the receptor and in doing so will prevent (or inhibit) the action of the agonist. To overcome the effect of a competitive antagonist, the probability of the agonist acting on the receptor needs to be increased, which can be done by increasing the concentration of the agonist.

**39** **Morphine is an** *agonist* **and naloxone is an** *antagonist* **of opiate receptors.**

Morphine is a agonist that acts on opiate receptors to cause a response in a cell. The effect of morphine can be blocked (or antagonized) by introducing the antagonist naloxone, which binds to the receptor and competes for the same binding site on the receptor so that morphine is less able to bind to the receptor and have a response.

**40** **Cyclizine is an** *antagonist* **of histamine, used to treat nausea and vomiting.**

Histamine receptors are found in an area of the brain that controls the feeling of nausea and vomiting. Inhibition of histamine in this area helps a patient to feel less nauseous. Cyclizine is an antagonist of H1 histamine receptors and by preventing the action of histamine in the vomiting centre of the brain it can prevent the feeling of nausea and vomiting.

**41** **A potent drug requires a** *lower* **concentration to bind to a receptor.**

Potency refers to the ability of the drug to activate a response and is related to the affinity of the drug for a receptor. The lower the concentration needed to produce that response, the more potent the drug is. This does not mean that a more potent drug is necessarily a better drug because it may not be very selective and may result in many side effects. If a drug is too potent, it may be easy to take too much drug and overdose.

**42** **In general, fat-soluble drugs cross cell** *membranes* **quicker than water-soluble drugs.**

Drugs that are fat soluble are lipophillic (liking the lipid environment and hating water, or hydrophobic). The cell membrane is a lipid environment that excludes water and charged particles. Fat-soluble drugs are not charged or ionized and are therefore not polar. They like the environment within the cell membrane and can easily pass into the cell membrane. Because the concentration of a drug will be high on one side of the membrane and low on the other side, the drug will pass from the side with a high concentration into the side with a low concentration easily and quickly using the lipid environment of the cell membrane and will not require a transport mechanism to cross the membrane.

**43** **The *liver* is the principal site of drug metabolism.**

Drug metabolism can occur in other tissues in the body, such as the lungs or plasma, depending on where the metabolic enzymes are located. The liver is the main site of drug metabolism because it contains large quantities of the enzymes involved in drug metabolism; in particular, the cytochrome P450 family of enzymes in Phase I metabolism, which are concentrated in the endoplasmic reticulum of hepatic cells. This gives the liver a large capacity to metabolize chemicals absorbed into the body.

**44** **Some drugs that *inhibit* drug metabolism can prolong the duration of action of drugs.**

When the body is constantly exposed to some drugs that are metabolized by the cytochrome P450 enzymes, the body can react by increasing the quantity of enzymes present in the liver. By increasing the capacity of the enzymes to metabolize drugs, these are called inducers of drug metabolism. Other drugs can reduce the amount of the enzymes or directly inhibit the enzymes involved. Drugs that inhibit the enzymes reduce the ability of the body to metabolize drugs. If a drug is not metabolized, this leads to an increase in the concentration of the drug within the body and therefore the drug will have a prolonged duration of action because it will be present in the body at therapeutic levels for a longer time.

**45** **Older adults and neonates have different *pharmacokinetics* to young adults.**

At both ends of the age scale, drugs are handled slightly differently compared with healthy young adults. The neonatal gut does not function like that of an adult, which affects absorption. The blood–brain barrier of the neonate is not fully formed, which has consequences for drug distribution, and in addition the neonatal liver enzymes are not fully functional. In older adults, both kidney function and the size of the liver are reduced, leading to a reduced ability to clear drugs from the body. These two categories of patients therefore have different pharmacokinetics compared with young healthy adults.

# 7    Drug calculations

## INTRODUCTION

Since the Nursing and Midwifery Council (NMC) introduced the standards of proficiency for nurse and midwife prescribers in 2006, there has been a requirement for a numerical assessment of nurse prescribers. This particular assessment causes many students considerable anxiety, especially as it requires a pass mark of 100%. The test is similar to the types of calculation that we do in everyday life. When at the supermarket, we are bombarded with 'special' or 'two for one' offers. The consumer needs to assess whether the offer is a better deal than the normal pack sitting next to the offer on the shelf. There is a simple calculation to be made in order to work out the best deal. In their professional life, prescribers need to be able to make similar simple calculations about drug doses and amounts in their everyday work.

We encourage students who have difficulty with numeracy to gain a confidence with numbers by practising as much as possible before the numeracy test. This chapter provides some arithmetic examples for students to gain the confidence needed to attempt the numeracy assessment. If more support is needed to gain that confidence with numbers, we recommend consulting a companion book in this series, *Nurses! Test Yourself in Essential Calculation Skills*. It will provide the formulae required for calculating different types of drug-related calculations and worked examples to help gain confidence.

> **Useful resources**
>
> Rogers, K.M.A. and Scott, W.N. (2011) *Nurses! Test Yourself in Essential Calculation Skills*. Maidenhead: Open University Press.
>
> TestandCalc is a web resource for health professionals to help with drug calculations: http://www.testandcalc.com.

# ROUNDING

With modern calculators, a simple calculation can result in a number that has eight or more digits in the answer (e.g. 0.123456789). Most of the numbers to the right of the decimal point are irrelevant in everyday situations, since we cannot measure things that accurately. To make the numbers more usable, we need to round the number up or down according to standard convention. If the number to the right of the decimal place is four or less, the number is left unchanged. However, if the number to the right of the decimal place is 5 or above, then one is added to the required decimal place. The number is then shortened, leaving only the required decimal places.

## WORKED EXAMPLE: ROUNDING

Round the following number to two decimal places:

2.37815

Second decimal place ↓

2.37     815
↑ Third decimal place

Add one to the second decimal place and delete the irrelevant digits:

The answer is **2.38**

Round the following numbers up to the required number of decimal places:

**1**  22.364    to 2 decimal places

**2**  5.6947    to 3 decimal places

**3**  1.6821    to 1 decimal place

**4**  8.1294    to 2 decimal places

**5**  0.9821    to 2 decimal places

**6**  7.6149    to 3 decimal places

**7**  12.591    to 1 decimal place

**8**  4.1987    to 3 decimal places

**9**   9.9981      to 2 decimal places

**10**  45.909      to 2 decimal places

# UNITS

Units are important to know in any calculation. Without units, we cannot know what the numbers mean. Do the numbers from a calculation indicate a volume, a mass, pounds sterling or elephants? The units therefore put a context to the calculation and indicate what the numbers mean. Unfortunately, we often forget to put the units in when we do calculations, because it is obvious to us what they are, but when communicating the numbers to other people, misunderstandings can occur if the units are not communicated as well.

The standard units used today conform to a metric system, the Système International d'Unités (SI units), which is a common language in science and medicine. The basic units of measurement are the gram (g) for mass (weight), the litre (L) for volume, and the metre (m) for length. Multiples of these are given a prefix that is useful in reducing the numbers of noughts, so reducing the complexity of the numbers.

Table 7.1 lists some commonly used prefixes and numbers.

**11** Fill in the gaps in Table 7.1.

**Table 7.1 Some commonly used prefixes and numbers for SI units**

| Prefix | Number | Factor | Prefix | Number | Factor |
|---|---|---|---|---|---|
| Milli (m) | 0.001 | $10^{-3}$ | Kilo (k) | 1,000 | $10^3$ |
| Micro (μ or mcg) | 0.000001 | $10^{-6}$ | Mega (?) | 1,000,000 | 10? |
| Nano (n) | ? | $10^{-?}$ | Giga (?) | ? | 10? |
| Pico (p) | ? | $10^{-?}$ | Tera (?) | ? | 10? |

Converting one unit into another requires moving the decimal place in the correct direction. A common mistake is to move the decimal place in the wrong direction, thus creating an error in the conversion.

Convert the following:

**12** 1500 millilitres to microlitres

**13** 378 microlitres to millilitres

**14**   20 microlitres to millilitres

**15**   0.75 millilitres to microlitres

**16**   0.4 grams to milligrams

**17**   1.11 kilograms to grams

**18**   193 micrograms to milligrams

**19**   800 metres to kilometres

**20**   1500 millimetres to metres

**21**   175,000 millimetres to kilometres

# PERCENTAGES

Convert the following into percentages:

**22**  0.56

**23**  0.43

**24**  0.034

**25**  1.42

Calculate the following:

**26**  20% of 23 × 17

**27**  65% of 27.4 × 11

**28**  2.3% of 56

**29**  16% of 87 ÷ 12

**30**  8% of (7 × 15) ÷ 3

**31** | 20% of $(1.5 \times 3) \div (3 \div 0.7)$

Drug strengths can be expressed in several ways.

# Percentage concentrations

There are three ways that a percentage concentration can be expressed:

- weight by volume (w/v)
- weight by weight (w/w)
- volume by volume (v/v)

The weight by volume (w/v) is the most common form of percentage concentration, and is used in particular with fluids and electrolytes. It indicates how much of the solid chemical is dissolved in the liquid. For example, 0.9% sodium chloride w/v means that 0.9 of a gram of NaCl was dissolved in a 100 mL volume of water.

# Concentrations in mg/mL

This is a common way to express drug concentrations. It is similar to w/v except that it gives a defined number of milligram per millilitre instead of per 100 mL.

# Concentrations in ratio strengths

These are used occasionally as '1 in $x$', for instance, 1 in 10,000, which means 1 gram in however many millilitres (in this case 10,000 mL).

# Concentration in units

Drugs such as heparin or insulin are measured in International Units (IU). Where a substance is extracted from an animal product or from a biosynthetic derivative, the purity of the drugs can vary. The IU is a measure of the biological activity of the drug.

# Concentration in molarity and molar solutions

This is based on the number of molecules of the drug dissolved in a litre of the solution. The mass of the drug depends on the overall chemical composition of the substance.

## DOSAGES

**32** Your patient requires a repeat prescription of Drug D, 125 micrograms twice a day. How many milligrams of drug will the patient receive in one week?

**33** You are nursing a terminally ill patient who requires a laxative suspension. You administer 20 mL of a 200 mg/5 mL preparation, once a day. How many grams of the laxative are given in one dose?

**34** Your patient has been prescribed 500 mg of a drug four times a day for two weeks. You have stocks of 250 mg tablets. How many tablets in total need to be supplied?

**35** You have given 25 mL of an antibiotic solution to your patient. The preparation comes at a concentration of 50 mg/mL. How many grams of antibiotic have you given to the patient?

**36** A child needs 350 mg of Drug P. You have an oral suspension of 120 mg/5 mL. What volume do you give the child? Give the answer correct to two decimal places.

**37** A patient is taking a diuretic for acute oedema. A total of 500 mg is required in 24 hours. The preparation is available in a 25 mg/5 mL solution. How many millilitres of solution are needed for the 24-hour period?

**38** You are asked to check a colleague's calculation. The drug is available in ampoules that contain 600 µg/mL. The nurse is about to give 1.25 mL to the patient. How many milligrams are they about to give the patient?

**39**  You prescribe a 1.5 g loading dose of an antibiotic suspension. The antibiotic comes as a concentration of 50 mg/mL. How many millilitres are required?

**40**  You have given a patient 0.55 mL of a solution that contains 5 mg/2 mL. How many milligrams of the drug have you administered?

**41**  You have prescribed a dose of 750 mg of Drug A to your patient. You have a solution that contains 250 mg/5 mL of the drug. Calculate the volume required to give the correct dose.

# DOSAGE BASED ON BODY WEIGHT

**42** You assess that a child requires Drug B as the treatment in two doses. The recommended daily dose is 25 mg/kg/day. Your child weighs 20 kg. How many milligrams are required for each dose?

**43** You have just given 10 mL of a solution that contains 150 mg/5 mL of Drug D to a child who weighs 12.5 kg. How many mg/kg have you given the child?

**44** Your colleague has just given 7 mL of a solution that contains 75 mg/2 mL of Drug E to a child who weighs 17.5 kg. How many mg/kg have been given to the child?

**45** A child of two and a half years weighs 13 kg and is prescribed Drug A at the recommended dose of 15 mg/kg/day. You have a stock solution at a concentration of 120 mg/5 mL. How many millilitres of the solution will give the recommended daily dose? Give your answer correct to one decimal place.

**46** An 80 kg man requires a 50 µg/kg dose of Drug J to reverse the effects of another drug. Drug J is stocked at 2.5 mg/mL. How many millilitres should be given to the patient?

**47** You have given a patient 0.5 mL of a solution that contains 1 mg/2 mL of a drug. The patient weighs 82 kg. How many µg/kg of the drug have you given the patient? Give your answer correct to one decimal place.

**48** A 75 kg person requires 70 µg/kg of Drug S. The drug is stocked at 2.5 mg/kg. What volume should be given to the patient?

**49** A patient weighing 83 kg is prescribed Drug T. The recommended dose is 50 μg/kg/day. You have the drug at a concentration of 2 mg/mL. How many millilitres should be given in a 24-hour period?

# RATES

**50** You are asked to set an infusion of 100 units of Drug M in 250 mL of normal saline. The prescribed dose for your patient is 10 units/hour. Calculate the hourly flow rate.

**51** A syringe contains 50 mL of an analgesic at a concentration of 5 mg/mL. If the flow rate is 2 mL/minute, how many milligrams have been given in 20 minutes?

**52** An infusion of 720 mg of Drug G is to be given over 24 hours. You have a solution of 5 mg/mL. How many mL/hour do you need to give the required dose?

**53** A patient is to receive an increase in the dose of a drug given by infusion. They are currently receiving an infusion of 5 mL/hour of a 20 µg/mL solution. They have been prescribed a dose of 3.6 mg/24 hours. By how much should you increase the infusion rate to the patient?

# ANSWERS

## ROUNDING

| 1 | 22.36 |

| 2 | 5.695 |

| 3 | 1.7 |

| 4 | 8.13 |

| 5 | 0.98 |

| 6 | 7.615 |

| 7 | 12.6 |

| 8 | 4.199 |

| 9 | 10.00 |

| 10 | 45.91 |

## UNITS

11

**Table 7.1 Some commonly used prefixes and numbers for SI units**

| Prefix | Number | Factor | Prefix | Number | Factor |
|--------|--------|--------|--------|--------|--------|
| Milli (m) | 0.001 | $10^{-3}$ | Kilo (k) | 1,000 | $10^3$ |
| Micro (μ or mcg) | 0.000 001 | $10^{-6}$ | Mega (M) | 1,000,000 | $10^6$ |
| Nano (n) | 0.000 000 001 | $10^{-9}$ | Giga (G) | 1,000,000,000 | $10^9$ |
| Pico (p) | 0.000 000 000 001 | $10^{-12}$ | Tera (T) | 1,000,000,000,000 | $10^{12}$ |

12  1,500,000 μL

13  0.378 mL

14  0.02 mL

15  750 μL

16  400 mg

17  1,110 g

18  0.193 mg

| 19 | 0.8 km |

| 20 | 1.5 m |

| 21 | 0.175 km |

## PERCENTAGES

| 22 | 56% |

| 23 | 43% |

| 24 | 3.4% |

| 25 | 142% |

| 26 | 78.2 |

| 27 | 195.91 |

| 28 | 1.288 |

| 29 | 1.16 |

30  2.8

31  0.21

## DOSAGES

32  1.75 mg

33  0.8 g

34  112 tablets

35  1.25 g

36  14.58 mL

37  100 mL

38  0.75 mg

39  30 mL

40  1.375 mg

**41** 15 mL

## DOSAGE BASED ON BODY WEIGHT

**42** 250 mg

**43** 24 mg/kg

**44** 15 mg/kg

**45** 8.1 mL

**46** 1.6 mL

**47** 3.0 µg/kg

**48** 2.1 mL

**49** 2.075 mL

## RATES

**50** 25 mL/hour

**51** 200 mg

**52** 6 mL/hour

**53** 2.5 mL/hour

# 8 Consultation skills and clinical decision making

## INTRODUCTION

The ability to take an accurate medical history from a patient and then synthesize the information obtained are key to being able to make an accurate diagnosis and subsequently to manage a diagnosis appropriately. Indeed, it could be argued that if we do not have the skills to obtain the information, how can we be sure of the diagnosis and therefore the treatment of the patient? The consultation influences the precision of the diagnosis and we know that effective history taking is essential, providing over 80% of diagnostic information (Silverman et al., 2004).

The success of the consultation depends not only on the content of the questioning but also on the process, i.e. *how* we undertake the consultation (Silverman et al., 2004). Therefore, more emphasis is now placed on the nurse–patient relationship – the rapport between the two and the communication skills used to obtain the information required. The patient needs to feel at ease and believe that their concerns and problems have been understood and respected. The patient also needs to reach a shared understanding with the nurse about the causes and management of their problems. This shared understanding is vital in ensuring concordance with any management plan suggested and particularly in optimizing medicines adherence (which we address in a later chapter). It is also important to note, however, that a nurse has a number of tasks to undertake to meet their agenda within the consultation. Thus a structured approach is vital in maximizing the efficiency and effectiveness of this process.

Many models of consultation exist, but the more recent ones note the importance of patient-centred care and the positive impact this has on patient satisfaction, improved outcomes, greater patient concordance/adherence, and nurses' job satisfaction. This chapter will test your knowledge on communication skills, in particular looking at consultation models, including the Calgary-Cambridge and Disease-Illness models. It will also test your knowledge on the structure of the consultation and will touch on decision-making models used in the diagnostic reasoning process (although therapeutic decision making is covered in Chapter 9). A sound understanding of these topics is vital if you are to be able to demonstrate competence in deciding when and if to prescribe as well as what to prescribe.

**Useful resources**

Thompson, C. and Dowding, D. (2002) *Clinical Decision Making and Judgement in Nursing.* London: Churchill Livingstone.

Skillscascade.com

## TRUE OR FALSE?

Are the following statements true or false?

**1** There are three types of consultation communication skills: content, process, and perceptual.

**2** One aid to effective listening is comfortable seating.

**3** Overly identifying with a patient's problem can be a sign of transference.

**4** All prescribers must make assessments and undertake prescribing decisions regularly to maintain registration.

**5** The Nursing and Midwifery Council (NMC) states that all nurses must have undertaken consultation skills/history taking training before being eligible for the NMP course.

**6** Closed questions are questions that cannot be answered with a simple 'yes' or 'no', or single-word answers.

**7** Non-verbal messages can be communicated by how someone dresses.

**8** Silence is an example of a paralinguistic feature of communication.

**9** Effective communication improves patient outcomes and increases clinician's job satisfaction.

**10** A paternalistic consultation style enhances concordance and patient-centred care.

# MULTIPLE CHOICE

Identify one correct answer for each of the following.

**11** Cue acquisition is:

a) data gathering

b) hypothesis formulation

c) observable body language

d) non-verbal communication

**12** Paralinguistic aspects of communication involve:

a) eye contact

b) posture

c) tone of voice

d) touch

**13** The NMC assesses competency to maintain NMP registration through:

a) number of prescriptions written by the nurse

b) number of patient consultations undertaken by the nurse

c) Post Registration Education and Practice (PREP)

d) proof of attendance at NMP update sessions

**14** Kinaesthetic cues are indicators of mental states that involve:

a) hearing

b) seeing

c) touching

d) moving

**15** When consulting with a patient whose first language is not English, the most appropriate person to interpret would be:

a) close family member

b) interpreter

c) health professional who speaks the same language

d) the person the patient brought with them to the consultation


**16** The humanistic psychologist John Heron developed a simple but effective model for use in consultations known as:

a) Calgary-Cambridge

b) Transactional Analysis

c) the Inner Consultation

d) Six-Category Intervention Analysis


**17** The unconscious projection of feelings or attitudes from patient to nurse is an example of:

a) transference

b) counter-transference

c) displacement

d) mirroring


**18** In decision making, heuristics can also be defined as:

a) 'rules of processing'

b) 'rules of intuition'

c) 'rules of thumb'

d) 'rules of cognition'

**19** Direct automatic retrieval of information from a well-organized knowledge base is an example of which clinical decision-making model?

a) hypothetico-deductive reasoning

b) pattern matching

c) collaborative reasoning

d) cognitive continuum

**20** Which of the following is *not* a barrier to effective communication?

a) third party

b) tiredness

c) confidentiality issues

d) attention focused 'out' rather than 'in'

# MATCH THE TERMS

Match each term with the correct description:

   **A.** summarizing
   **B.** facilitative responses
   **C.** signposting
   **D.** hypothetico-deductive reasoning
   **E.** metacognition
   **F.** narrative reasoning
   **G.** cognitive processing

**21** The thought processes used when making a judgement or decision.

**22** Structures the consultation, helps to use time constructively, and reduces uncertainty for both the patient and the nurse.

**23** Understanding the patient's perspective/experience of their illness.

**24** Transitional statement that allows the doctor to signal a change in direction, and move from one section of the consultation to another.

**25** Words or actions that encourage the patient to talk.

**26** A form of problem solving starting with a prediction about variables that might affect an outcome, from which it is possible to form logical, testable conclusions.

**27** Self-awareness, self-monitoring, and reflective processes.

# FILL IN THE BLANKS

Fill in the blanks in each statement using the options in the box.
*Not all of them are required, so choose carefully!*

| | |
|---|---|
| gathering | medication |
| assessment | closing |
| action | accessing |
| conscious | immediate |
| hypotheses | limited |
| communicate | open |
| who | delayed |
| what | planning |
| comprehensive | accessible |
| prescriber | how |

**28** The mnemonic 2-WHAM is a useful tool to help nurses prescribe the most appropriate product. This stands for:

W- _____ is it for?

W- _____ are the symptoms?

H-_____ long have the symptoms been present?

A- _____ taken so far.

M- _____ currently being taken.

**29** The Calgary-Cambridge Model of consultation has four main areas in its structure: (a) initiating the session, (b) information _____, (c) explanation and _____, and (d) _____ the session.

**30** The NMC states that you have a responsibility to _____ effectively with other practitioners involved in the care of the patient/client. You must refer the patient/client to another _____ when it is necessary to do so.

**31** In order to prescribe for a patient/client, you must satisfy yourself that you have undertaken a full _____ of the patient/client, including taking a thorough history and, where possible, _____ a full clinical record.

**32** Hypothetico-deductive reasoning can be defined as a process of generating a _____ number of _____ early in the encounter and using them to guide the subsequent data collection.

**33** According to the NMC, nurse prescribers should ensure records are accurate, _____, contemporaneous, and _____ by all members of a prescribing team (effective policies must be in place locally to enable this to happen).

**34** One view of intuition defines it as the _____ knowing of something without the _____ use of reason.

**LABELLING EXERCISE**

Add the labels in the box to Figure 8.1.

| | |
|---|---|
| Love/belonging needs | Physiological needs |
| Self-actualization | Safety needs |
| Esteem needs | |

**Figure 8.1  Maslow's (1970) hierarchy of needs**

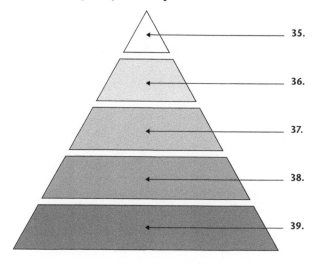

35.

36.

37.

38.

39.

# ANSWERS

## TRUE OR FALSE?

**1** | **There are three types of consultation communication skills: content, process, and perceptual.**

Content skills relate to the substance of what the nurse says, process skills are how they communicate, and perceptual skills relate to internal decision making, thoughts, and feelings during the communication episode.

**2** | **One aid to effective listening is comfortable seating.**

The comfort of both patient and nurse has been found to have an effect on how well people actually listen. When we are uncomfortable our focus becomes 'inward', often linked to internal dialogue. When we have no distractions, our focus is 'outward', which aids 'active listening'.

**3** | **Overly identifying with a patient's problem can be a sign of transference.**

This is a sign of counter-transference, the unconscious process whereby the nurse responds to the patient in a manner similar to a significant past relationship. Other signs include:

   i.    not listening attentively

   ii.   interpreting too soon

   iii.  misjudging the patient's level of feeling

   iv.  becoming too active in giving advice

   v.    becoming overly identified with the patient's problem

   vi.  gaining vicarious pleasure in the patient's story

   vii. engaging in power struggles with the patient

   viii. running late, running over time or covering the same material with the patient over and over again

**4** | **All prescribers must make assessments and undertake prescribing decisions regularly to maintain registration.**

It is the nurse's responsibility to update their knowledge and skills, so enabling him or her to prescribe competently and safely. As a nurse or midwife who is recorded on the register as being a prescriber, he or she should ensure that continuing professional development is in line with their role as a prescriber.

**5** **The Nursing and Midwifery Council (NMC) states that all nurses must have undertaken consultation skills/history taking training before being eligible for the NMP course.**

The NMC requires employers to undertake an appraisal of a registrant's suitability to prescribe before they apply for a training place. Where the registrant is not undertaking a module to prepare them in diagnosis and physical assessment alongside the nurse/midwife independent/ supplementary prescribing programme, then the employer is responsible for confirming that the applicant has been assessed as competent to take a history, undertake a clinical assessment, and diagnose before being put forward. Employers should not put registrants forward if they have not demonstrated the ability to diagnose in their area of speciality.

**6** **Closed questions are questions that cannot be answered with a simple 'yes' or 'no', or single-word answers.**

Closed questions do not allow for any explanation to be added. For example, asking 'Is it painful?' will result in a 'yes/no' answer, whereas asking an open question such as 'Can you describe the pain?' will result in the patient describing the pain they are experiencing. In general, open questions allow for a more detailed disclosure; however, it must be remembered that closed questions have their uses, particularly when the nurse wishes to clarify certain points.

**7** **Non-verbal messages can be communicated by how someone dresses.**

The way in which we dress can provide vital cues as to how we wish to be viewed but can also be related to emotion and culture as well as giving strong messages to those we come into contact with. Whether we do this consciously or unconsciously, it still communicates non-verbally to those around us.

**8** **Silence is an example of a paralinguistic feature of communication.**

Paralinguistics is the study of speech and is a form of non-verbal communication. Paralinguistic cues involve volume (Is the voice low or is it loud when speaking? Does the person appear confident, sad, happy or angry?), pitch, inflection/tone (inflection is the variation in the change of pitch to create meaning), speed (rate of speech), intensity (humour, monotony, anger, sadness), silence (emphasizing a point or asking a question and using silence to generate impact to the spoken word), and quality.

**9** **Effective communication improves patient outcomes and increases clinician's job satisfaction.**

Research into patient–provider communication has established that effective communication has benefits for both patients and healthcare professionals alike. Generally speaking, the benefits include improved patient outcomes, a reduction in complaints/litigation, and fewer clinical errors.

**10** **A paternalistic consultation style enhances concordance and patient-centred care.**

Paternalism suggests a style of communication whereby the clinician makes decisions based on what he or she thinks is in the best interests of the patient, whereas patient-centred care requires a collaborative approach with active participation from both clinician and patient. Research suggests that the latter is better for improving concordance issues in prescribing.

 **MULTIPLE CHOICE**
Correct answers identified in bold italics.

**11** **Cue acquisition is:**

a) *data gathering*  b) hypothesis formulation

c) observable body language  d) non-verbal communication

Cue acquisition is the information gathered from verbal and non-verbal information identified.

**12** **Paralinguistic aspects of communication involve:**

a) eye contact  b) posture  *c) tone of voice*  d) touch

Paralinguistics refers to vocal communication that is separate from actual language. This includes factors such as tone of voice, loudness, inflection, and pitch.

**13** **The NMC assesses competency to maintain NMP registration through:**

a)  number of prescriptions written by the nurse

b)  number of patient consultations undertaken by the nurse

c)  *Post Registration Education and Practice (PREP)*

d)  proof of attendance at NMP update sessions

In the UK, the registration of nurses, midwives, and specialist community public health nurses is a prerequisite of their employment as registered practitioners. As prescribing is a registerable qualification by the NMC, PREP covers this area of nurses' competence along with general fitness to practise.

**14** **Kinaesthetic cues are indicators of mental states that involve:**

a) hearing   b) seeing   c) touching   *d) moving*

Kinaesthetics describes feedback from the body that gives an individual an awareness of their bodily position in space. Kinaesthetic cues are those cues that involve information that is gathered from observing the movement of another person. Cues such as posture, distance, touch, gestures, breathing rate, and muscle tone are all examples of kinaesthetic cues and can give vital information about the thoughts and feelings of the patient.

**15** **When consulting with a patient whose first language is not English, the most appropriate person to interpret would be:**

a)  close family member

*b)  interpreter*

c)  health professional who speaks the same language

d)  the person the patient brought with them to the consultation

It is always best practice, wherever possible, to use an interpreter who has had time to build rapport with the patient. The ideal interpreter is a neutral, objective person familiar with both languages and cultures. Family members are more likely to distort meanings and may present confidentiality conflicts for both patient and nurse. If you do use an interpreter, make sure you still direct your consultation to the patient and keep questions short and clear.

**16** **The humanistic psychologist John Heron developed a simple but effective model for use in consultations known as:**

a)  Calgary-Cambridge

b)  Transactional Analysis

c)  the Inner Consultation

*d)  Six-Category Intervention Analysis*

Within an overall setting of patient-centredness, the nurse's interventions fall within six categories:

i.   Prescriptive – giving advice or instructions

ii.  Informative – imparting new knowledge, instructing or interpreting

iii. Confronting – challenging a restrictive attitude or behaviour, giving direct feedback within a caring context

iv.  Cathartic – seeking to release emotion in the form of weeping, laughter, trembling or anger

v.   Catalytic – encouraging the patient to discover and explore their own latent thoughts and feelings

vi.  Supportive – offering comfort and approval, affirming the patient's intrinsic value.

Heron saw each category as having clear functions within the consultation, and by identifying how patients communicate and then responding with the appropriate intervention, communication is enhanced.

**17** **The unconscious projection of feelings or attitudes from patient to nurse is an example of:**

*a) transference*   b) counter-transference   c) displacement
d) mirroring

First described by Sigmund Freud, consultations can be influenced by this phenomenon whereby the patient unconsciously projects onto the nurse thoughts, behaviours, and emotional reactions: feelings of love, hate, ambivalence, and dependency. The closer the attachment in the patient–nurse relationship, the more likely is transference to occur. Although it is often viewed as a negative influence, it can help build a connection between the patient and nurse as long as the nurse identifies it. Knowledge of the patient's transference reaction may or may not assist us in understanding how the patient experiences his or her world and how past relationships influence current behaviour.

**18** **In decision making, heuristics can also be defined as:**

a) 'rules of processing'   b) 'rules of intuition'   *c) 'rules of thumb'*
d) 'rules of cognition'

These are particular strategies that individuals develop to process a large amount of information efficiently. They bypass having to process a large amount of irrelevant data when making judgements and decisions.

**19** **Direct automatic retrieval of information from a well-organized knowledge base is an example of which clinical decision-making model?**

a) hypothetico-deductive reasoning   *b) pattern matching*
c) collaborative reasoning   d) cognitive continuum

Experienced healthcare professionals are more likely to use a process of 'pattern matching', which involves recognizing similarities between the patient being considered and others encountered in the past.

**20** **Which of the following is *not* a barrier to effective communication?**

a) third party   b) tiredness   c) confidentiality issues
*d) attention focused 'out' rather than 'in'*

Focusing the attention 'out' rather than 'in' helps the clinician to utilize active listening, thus improving communication. A barrier to effective communication would be focusing attention 'in', such as focusing on internal dialogue rather than the patient's story.

## MATCH THE TERMS

**21** The thought processes used when making a judgement or decision.

**G.** cognitive processing

**22** Structures the consultation, helps to use time constructively, and reduces uncertainty for both the patient and the nurse.

**A.** summarizing

**23** Understanding the patient's perspective/ experience of their illness.

**F.** narrative reasoning

**24** Transitional statement that allows the doctor to signal a change in direction, and move from one section of the consultation to another.

**C.** signposting

**25** Words or actions that encourage the patient to talk.

**B.** facilitative responses

**26** A form of problem solving starting with a prediction about variables that might affect an outcome, from which it is possible to form logical, testable conclusions.

**D.** hypothetico-deductive reasoning

**27** Self-awareness, self-monitoring, and reflective processes.

**E.** metacognition

## FILL IN THE BLANKS

**28** **2-WHAM stands for:**
- <u>Who</u> is it for?
- <u>What</u> are the symptoms?

- *How* long have the symptoms been present?
- *Action* taken so far.
- *Medication* currently being taken.

The mnemonic **2-WHAM** is used by community pharmacists as a template to assist them when recommending over-the-counter (OTC) therapies. However, it is a useful template for all health professionals and can help minimize the chance of error.

**29** **The Calgary-Cambridge Model of consultation has four main areas in its structure: (a) initiating the session, (b) information _gathering_, (c) explanation and _planning_, and (d) _closing_ the session.**

Many consultation models have been developed over the years. Suzanne Kurtz and Jonathan Silverman developed a model of the consultation, encapsulated within a practical teaching tool, known as the Calgary-Cambridge Observation Guides. The Guides define the content of a communication skills curriculum by delineating and structuring the skills that have been shown by research and theory to aid clinician–patient communication.

**30** **The NMC states that you have a responsibility to _communicate_ effectively with other practitioners involved in the care of the patient/client. You must refer the patient/client to another _prescriber_ when it is necessary to do so.**

Communication and interpersonal skills are essential components in delivering quality nursing care. Communication is identified as an essential skill that nurses require and has been demonstrated to improve patient outcomes. This communication is as important when dealing with other practitioners as when dealing with patients/clients themselves.

**31** **In order to prescribe for a patient/client, you must satisfy yourself that you have undertaken a full _assessment_ of the patient/client, including taking a thorough history and, where possible, _accessing_ a full clinical record.**

Prescribers are accountable for their decision to prescribe and must therefore be able to demonstrate that they have undertaken a full assessment of the patient in order to inform their prescribing decision.

**32** **Hypothetico-deductive reasoning can be defined as a process of generating a _limited_ number of _hypotheses_ early in the encounter and using them to guide the subsequent data collection.**

Hypothetico-deductive reasoning involves starting with a general theory of all possible factors that might affect an outcome and forming a hypothesis; then deductions are made from that hypothesis to predict what the specific outcome might be.

**33** **According to the NMC, nurse prescribers should ensure records are accurate, _comprehensive_, contemporaneous, and _accessible_ by all members of a prescribing team (effective policies must be in place locally to enable this to happen).**

Records should include the prescription details, together with relevant details of the consultation with the patient/client. The maximum time allowed between writing the prescription and entering the details into the general record should not exceed 48 hours.

**34** **One view of intuition defines it as the _immediate_ knowing of something without the _conscious_ use of reason.**

There are some differences in the way intuition is defined in the literature, but there is also a fair degree of agreement in that most definitions include rapid perception, lack of awareness of the processes engaged, concomitant presence of emotions, and holistic understanding of the problem situation.

## LABELLING EXERCISE

Add the labels in the box to Figure 8.1.

**Figure 8.1 Maslow's (1970) hierarchy of needs**

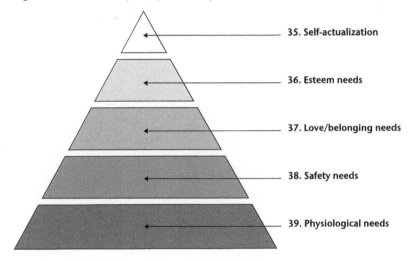

35. Self-actualization

36. Esteem needs

37. Love/belonging needs

38. Safety needs

39. Physiological needs

# 9 Therapeutic decision making and principles of safe prescribing

## INTRODUCTION

As nurse prescribers we are legally and ethically bound to ensure that any treatment we use to manage a patient's condition is evidence-based and effective, while keeping risk to a minimum, ensuring cost-effectiveness and, most importantly, respecting the patient's wishes. Unfortunately, this can be a difficult task and ensuring maximum effectiveness of a medication can sometimes incur greater risk to our patients. Therapeutic decision making is about balancing these influences and coming to a decision; weighing up the benefits against the risks and ensuring joint decision making so as to maximize the chances of adherence. To do this we need to be thorough in our history taking, in particular ensuring we have understood our patient's perspective and that we have all the information necessary to be able to make that decision. A detailed drug history is imperative as well as ensuring we have details of allergies and what effects these have on our patients. This helps us not to prescribe anything that may interact with current medication, helps identify a possible allergic reaction, and also helps to prevent the prescribing of a medication that will cause harm to our patients.

Other factors can impact on this already complex process and we need to be cognisant of these and ensure we have strategies to deal with them before they occur. For example, our colleagues may view our ability to prescribe as a way around difficulties in their own prescribing practice, or friends and family members may ask us for prescriptions. What is legal and ethical is paramount to the safety of our patients and our overall prescribing practice.

---

**Useful resources**

Nursing and Midwifery Council
www.nmc-uk.org

UK Medicines Information
www.ukmi.nhs.uk

## TRUE OR FALSE?

Are the following statements true or false?

**1** Once registered as a nurse independent prescriber, that nurse can prescribe medications for patients who have been assessed by their colleagues.

**2** Prescribing for a relative who is not your patient should be avoided.

**3** Once you have passed the non-medical prescribing course and have had your results confirmed, you can start prescribing immediately.

**4** If you issue a repeat prescription for a patient, the person who assessed and diagnosed the condition that required medication is accountable for that prescribing decision.

**5** Prescribing by telephone or in other non-face-to-face situations is not acceptable.

**6** It is acceptable for a pharmacist to dispense an emergency supply of medication to a patient based on information from a prescriber without having a suitable prescription in their possession.

**7** You may prescribe a controlled drug for someone close to you only if no other person with the legal right to prescribe is available.

**8** Computer-generated signatures on computer-generated prescriptions may be used providing appropriate software is available.

**9** All prescriptions are valid for 6 months.

**10** You may delegate administration of a medication that you have prescribed.

**MULTIPLE CHOICE**

Identify one correct answer for each of the following.

**11** Which information is a legal requirement on a prescription for a child under 12 years?

a) height

b) weight

c) age

d) all of the above

**12** Which of the following would be least likely to cause error because of the way it is written?

a) Chlorpheniramine maleate 4.0 mg every 4–6 hrs prn. Max 24.0 mg daily

b) Chlorpheniramine maleate 4 mg one tablet qds prn. Max 24 mg in 24 hours

c) Chlorpheniramine maleate 4 mg one tablet every 4–6 hours. Max 24 mg in 24 hours

d) Chlorpheniramine maleate 4 mg 4–6 hourly as required. Max 24 mg

**13** To be valid, a prescription for an adult must:

a) be written in indelible ink

b) be hand-written

c) include the patient's age

d) include the name of the patient's registered general practitioner

**14** When writing supplementary warnings of advice on a prescription, these should not:

a) be written as numerical codes

b) be in line with warnings or advice in the British National Formulary (BNF)

c) be written in full

d) be written underneath the prescribed medication but should be written on the strip of paper on the side of the FP10

**15** When prescribing controlled drugs, this must never:

a) be pre-written by anyone other than the prescriber

b) be altered in any way by the pharmacist

c) be written on a private prescription

d) be dispensed unless all the information is complete

**16** The most common drug error is:

a) administering the wrong dose

b) administering the wrong medication

c) administering the medication via the wrong route

d) administering a medication that the patient is allergic to

**17** Each year, medication errors in the UK are responsible for approximately:

a) 5,000 deaths

b) 6,000 deaths

c) 7,000 deaths

d) 8,000 deaths

**18** The costs associated with adverse events and inappropriate prescribing have been estimated at more than

a) £550 million per year

b) £650 million per year

c) £750 million per year

d) £850 million per year

**19** In primary care, the rate of prescribing errors has been estimated to be:

a) 5%

b) 10–11%

c) 15%

d) 20%

**20** To keep blank prescription pads secure, they should always:

a) be used by one prescriber only

b) be locked away when not in use

c) be stored and used in the order pertaining to the numerical sequence written on each prescription

d) all of the above

**MATCH THE TERMS**

Match each term with the correct description.

- **A.** competence
- **B.** accountable
- **C.** dispense
- **D.** administer
- **E.** patient group direction (PGD)
- **F.** patient specific direction (PSD)
- **G.** pharmacy medicine (P)

**21** Medicines that can only be sold through a registered pharmacy under the personal supervision of a pharmacist.

**22** To give a substance to a patient via a certain route.

**23** The state or quality of being adequately or well qualified.

**24** Required or expected to justify actions or decisions.

**25** A written instruction from a doctor, dentist or nurse prescriber for a medicine to be supplied and/or administered to a named person.

**26** To label from stock and supply a clinically appropriate medicine to a patient usually against a written prescription.

**27** A written instruction for the supply or administration of named medicines to specific groups of patients.

# FILL IN THE BLANKS

Fill in the blanks in each statement using the options in the box.
*Not all of them are required, so choose carefully!*

| | |
|---|---|
| Schedules | oral |
| dated | indelible |
| name | 28 |
| tablets | practitioner |
| parenteral | days' |
| intravenous | |

**28** When writing a prescription, it must be written and signed in _____ ink by the _____ using their own name.

**29** The validity of any prescription for _____ 2, 3, and 4 CDs to be restricted to _____ days.

**30** For all prescriptions, either the number of _____ to be prescribed must be written on the prescription or the number of _____ treatment required in the box on the FP10.

**31** To avoid inadvertent intravenous administration of oral medicines, the appropriate syringe should be used. _____ syringes are not compatible with _____ or other _____ devices.

**32** Prescriptions should be _____, and should include the full _____ and address of the patient.

## LABELLING EXERCISE

Add the labels in the box to Figure 9.1.

| | |
|---|---|
| Record keeping | Strategy |
| Reflect | Negotiate 'contract' |
| Holistic assessment | Review |
| Consider product choice | |

**Figure 9.1 The prescribing pyramid (NPC, 1999). Each step should be considered carefully before the next is approached.**

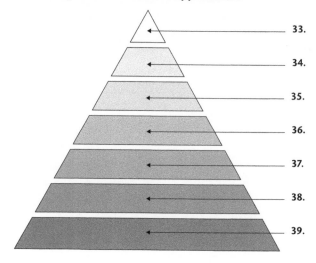

33.

34.

35.

36.

37.

38.

39.

## TRUE OR FALSE?

**1** Once registered as a nurse independent prescriber, that nurse can prescribe medications for patients who have been assessed by their colleagues.

The NMC recognizes that there are circumstances in which a nurse or midwife may be asked to prescribe on behalf of a colleague for a patient/ client they have not personally assessed. The NMC suggests, however, that wherever possible this should be avoided. Nurses and midwifes are accountable if they do decide to prescribe.

**2** Prescribing for a relative who is not your patient should be avoided.

The guidance from the NMC is that nurse prescribers should never prescribe for anyone with whom they have a close personal or emotional relationship unless under exceptional circumstances. It falls to the nurse prescriber to be able to justify what is considered 'exceptional'. The patient should be referred to another registered prescriber for assessment and management.

**3** Once you have passed the non-medical prescribing course and have had your results confirmed, you can start prescribing immediately.

You may only prescribe once you have successfully completed an NMC-approved programme, and recorded this in the NMC register. You also need to have the support and permission of your employer.

**4** If you issue a repeat prescription for a patient, the person who assessed and diagnosed the condition that required medication is accountable for that prescribing decision.

You may issue a repeat prescription, but you are responsible as the signatory of the prescription and are accountable for your practice. Before signing a repeat prescription, you must be satisfied that it is safe and appropriate to do so and that secure procedures are in place to ensure that the patient is issued with the right prescription and for the right condition. Thus you must satisfy yourself through a reassessment that the patient still requires the medication and that suitable provision is made for assessing and reviewing need.

**5** **Prescribing by telephone or in other non-face-to-face situations is not acceptable.**

It is acceptable for such prescribing to take place as long as the prescriber is able to undertake a *full* medical and drug history assessment, identifying the likely cause of the condition to be treated. They should also ensure there is sufficient justification for a prescribing decision, that the treatment and/or medicine is not contra-indicated for the patient, making a clear, accurate, legible and contemporaneous record of all medicines prescribed. Where these requirements cannot be met, prescribing should not be undertaken and the patient should be assessed by non-remote means.

**6** **It is acceptable for a pharmacist to dispense an emergency supply of medication to a patient based on information from a prescriber without having a suitable prescription in their possession.**

The pharmacist needs to be satisfied that the prescriber by means of some emergency is unable to provide a prescription immediately, that they undertake to issue one within 72 hours, that it is not a controlled drug, that the drug is supplied with *full* directions of the prescriber prescribing it, and that they make an entry into the prescription book with full details of the patient, prescriber, and drug and that the entry is updated once the prescription is received.

**7** **You may prescribe a controlled drug for someone close to you only if no other person with the legal right to prescribe is available.**

This is only applicable if that treatment is immediately necessary to save life, avoid significant deterioration in the patient's health or alleviate otherwise uncontrollable pain. You must be able to justify your actions and must document your relationship and the emergency circumstances that necessitated you prescribing a controlled drug for someone close to you.

**8** **Computer-generated signatures on computer-generated prescriptions may be used providing appropriate software is available.**

Computer-generated signatures do not meet the legal requirement for the prescription to be signed in ink personally by the prescriber. Computer-generated prescriptions may be used with appropriate software, but these must be signed in indelible ink, by the prescriber, preferably immediately after printing.

**9** **All prescriptions are valid for 6 months.**

Controlled drug prescriptions are only valid for 28 days; all other prescriptions are valid for 6 months.

**10** **You may delegate administration of a medication that you have prescribed.**

You remain accountable for your actions and you must be sure the person to whom you have delegated is competent and has received sufficient training to administer the prescribed medication. **Note:** You may not delegate administration of a medication that you supply/administer via a Patient Group Direction.

 **MULTIPLE CHOICE**

Correct answers identified in bold italics.

**11** **Which information is a legal requirement on a prescription for a child under 12 years?**

a) height   b) weight   *c) age*   d) all of the above

Including the age and date of birth of the patient on the prescription is good practice but it is a legal requirement for children under 12 years of age. Height is not required and weight is only used on prescriptions for babies.

**12** **Which of the following would be least likely to cause error because of the way it is written?**

a)  Chlorpheniramine maleate 4.0 mg every 4–6 hrs prn. Max 24.0 mg daily

b)  Chlorpheniramine maleate 4 mg one tablet qds prn. Max 24 mg in 24 hours

c)  *Chlorpheniramine maleate 4 mg one tablet every 4–6 hours. Max 24 mg in 24 hours*

d)  Chlorpheniramine maleate 4 mg 4–6 hourly as required. Max 24 mg

It is not good practice to use decimal points for whole numbers. Latin abbreviations may be used but this is not always specific and may be misinterpreted. Writing 'one tablet' is clearer for the patient and writing words in full leads to less chance of misunderstanding.

**13** **To be valid, a prescription for an adult must:**

a)  *be written in indelible ink*

b)  be hand-written

c)  include the patient's age

d)  include the name of the patient's registered general practitioner

The British National Formulary (BNF) states that indelible ink must be used for all prescriptions. Guidelines on the legal requirements for written prescriptions can be found at the beginning of the BNF.

**14** **When writing supplementary warnings of advice on a prescription, these should not:**

a) *be written as numerical codes*

b) be in line with warnings or advice in the British National Formulary (BNF)

c) be written in full

d) be written underneath the prescribed medication but should be written on the strip of paper on the side of the FP10.

It is important that this information is clear and written as per BNF instructions. These may change and must therefore be written in full sentences. It is not usually necessary to write warnings on a prescription, as usually the pharmacist will do this on the dispensing packaging for the patient.

**15** **When prescribing controlled drugs, this must never:**

a) be pre-written by anyone other than the prescriber

b) be altered in any way by the pharmacist

c) be written on a private prescription

d) *be dispensed unless all the information is complete*

Legal requirements state that full information must be provided.

**16** **The most common drug error is:**

a) *administering the wrong dose*

b) administering the wrong medication

c) administering the medication via the wrong route

d) administering a medication that the patient is allergic to

The most common types of drug errors resulting in patient death involve the wrong dose (40.9%), the wrong drug (16%), and the wrong route of administration (9.5%).

**17** **Each year, medication errors in the UK are responsible for approximately:**

a) 5,000 deaths    b) 6,000 deaths    *c) 7,000 deaths*    d) 8,000 deaths

The National Patient Safety Agency Report (2004) highlighted that medication errors were estimated to kill 7,000 patients per annum and account for nearly one in twenty hospital admissions.

**18** **The costs associated with adverse events and inappropriate prescribing have been estimated at more than**

a) £550 million per year
b) £650 million per year
*c)* *£750 million per year*
d) £850 million per year

Medication errors account for approximately 20% of all clinical negligence claims against doctors in both primary and secondary care. The costs associated with adverse events and inappropriate prescribing have been estimated at more than £750 million per year.

**19** **In primary care, the rate of prescribing errors has been estimated to be:**

a) 5%   *b) 10–11%*   c) 15%   d) 20%

In primary care, the rate of prescribing errors has been estimated to be 10–11%. Communication of prescribing information between primary and secondary care has also been shown to be less than ideal, as evidenced by a study which estimated that 50% of patients were failing to take the correct medicine one month after discharge.

**20** **In order to keep blank prescription pads secure, they should always:**

a) be used by one prescriber only
*b)* *be locked away when not in use*
c) be stored and used in the order pertaining to the numerical sequence written on each prescription
d) all of the above

It is also useful to record serial numbers of prescriptions as they are received and lock away any pads/prescriptions not in use. Generally speaking, it is safer to take only the number of prescriptions required rather than a whole pad if visiting patients at home, for example.

 **MATCH THE TERMS**

**21** Medicines that can only be sold through a registered pharmacy under the personal supervision of a pharmacist.    **G**. pharmacy medicine (P)

**22** To give a substance to a patient via a certain route.    **D**. administer

| 23 | The state or quality of being adequately or well qualified. | A. competence |
|---|---|---|
| 24 | Required or expected to justify actions or decisions. | B. accountable |
| 25 | A written instruction from a doctor, dentist or nurse prescriber for a medicine to be supplied and/or administered to a named person. | F. patient specific direction (PSD) |
| 26 | To label from stock and supply a clinically appropriate medicine to a patient usually against a written prescription. | C. dispense |
| 27 | A written instruction for the supply or administration of named medicines to specific groups of patients. | E. patient group direction (PGD) |

## FILL IN THE BLANKS

**28** **When writing a prescription, it must be written and signed in _indelible_ ink by the _practitioner_ using their own name.**

Many prescriptions are now computer-produced but, if you are hand-writing one, it must be written legibly in indelible ink, dated and stating the full name and address of the patient. All prescriptions should be signed by the independent prescriber whose name appears on the prescription. It should also contain their contact details and details of their NMC registration number.

**29** **The validity of any prescription for _Schedules_ 2, 3 and 4 CDs to be restricted to _28_ days.**

Changes following amendments to the Misuse of Drugs Regulations came into force in July 2006. These include:

- A new requirement that patients or others collecting medicines on their behalf must sign for them.

- Validity of any prescription for Schedules 2, 3 and 4 CDs to be restricted to 28 days.

- Strong recommendation that the maximum quantity be limited to 30 days for prescriptions of Schedules 2, 3 and 4 CDs.

**30** **For all prescriptions, either the number of *tablets* to be prescribed must be written on the prescription or the number of *days'* treatment required in the box on the FP10.**

It is good prescribing practice to state number of days treatment or number of tablets to be supplied when writing a prescription on an FP10. This helps to prevent drug errors and prescriptions being altered after medications have been prescribed. This information is also required for the pharmacist dispensing the medications.

**31** **To avoid inadvertent intravenous administration of oral medicines, the appropriate syringe should be used. *Oral* syringes are not compatible with *intravenous* or other *parenteral* devices.**

BNF guidance (2012) states 'To avoid inadvertent intravenous administration of oral liquid medicines, only an appropriate **oral** or **enteral syringe** should be used to measure an oral liquid medicine (if a medicine spoon or graduated measure cannot be used); these syringes should **not** be compatible with intravenous or other parenteral devices. Oral or enteral syringes should be clearly labeled "Oral" or "Enteral" in a large font size; it is the healthcare practitioner's responsibility to label the syringe with this information if the manufacturer has not done so.'

**32** **Prescriptions should be *dated*, and should include the full *name* and address of the patient.**

Again this is good prescribing practice and is necessary to help reduce the chance of error. Prescriptions should also include the date of birth and age of the patient, particularly for children under 12 years of age where it is a legal requirement to do so.

**LABELLING EXERCISE**

Add the labels in the box to Figure 9.1.

**Figure 9.1 The prescribing pyramid (NPC, 1999). Each step should be considered carefully before the next is approached.**

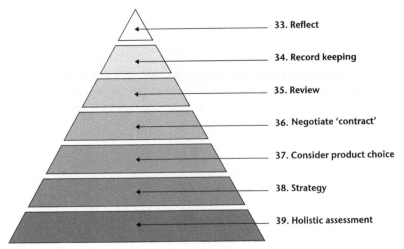

33. Reflect
34. Record keeping
35. Review
36. Negotiate 'contract'
37. Consider product choice
38. Strategy
39. Holistic assessment

# 10 Prescribing errors

## INTRODUCTION

Medicines are one of the most powerful tools to improve the health of patients, but when used inappropriately they are also harmful. Medication errors are perhaps the biggest preventable cause of harm to a patient. They can be defined as any error in the prescribing, dispensing or administration of a drug. In the UK, the prescribing error rate in primary care is approximately 7.5% with around one in fifteen admissions to hospital being related to medication problems (Garfield et al., 2009). Incorrect medicines or the doses given may occur as a result of choosing the wrong medicines, confusion over drug names, numerical errors or missing information. They generally fall into the three categories of slips, lapses or errors (Dean et al., 2002).

The aim of this chapter is to highlight when and where medication errors arise and to help the practitioner eliminate errors from their working practice. Some patients will be particularly vulnerable to these errors. It is therefore important to be aware of the drugs that pose the most risk to patients and how errors can be avoided.

> **Useful resources**
>
> National Prescribing Centre (2011) *10 Top Tips for GPs: Strategies for Safer Prescribing*. Liverpool: NICE. Available at: http://www.npc.co.uk/evidence/resources/10_top_tips_for_gps.pdf.

## TRUE OR FALSE?

Are the following statements true of false?

**1** Drugs that are most commonly associated with medication errors have a wide therapeutic index.

**2** More prescribing errors are made by prescribers when they are unfamiliar with the drugs they are prescribing.

**3** The majority of prescribing errors do not result in harm to the patient.

**4** When writing a prescription, abbreviations should be avoided.

**5** Poor writing can lead to administration errors.

**6** Drug administration errors often result when one of the 'five cardinal rights' of drug administration are not followed.

**7** It is usual when writing a drug dose to precede the decimal point with a zero and to leave out trailing zeros.

**8** Residents of care homes are particularly vulnerable to medication errors.

**MULTIPLE CHOICE**

Identify one correct answer for each of the following.

**9** Medication errors can be made by failing to check:

a) for allergies to the medication

b) for stocks in the pharmacy

c) directions on the packaging

d) the patient's date of birth

**10** Medication reviews ensure:

a) drug costs are reduced

b) contact with the patient is maintained

c) drug administration is correct

d) side effects are detected

**11** Communication problems with the patient can result in:

a) dispensing errors

b) fewer medicines to choose from

c) incorrect use of medication

d) improved safety of the patient

**12** When writing a prescription it is good practice:

a) to use Latin abbreviations

b) to assume that a previous drug dose is correct

c) to write units out in full

d) to abbreviate drug names

**MATCH THE TERMS**

Match each term with the correct description:

A. administration error

B. dispensing error

C. knowledge-related mistake

D. near miss

E. prescribing error

F. transcribing error

**13** Incorrect drug selection for the patient.

**14** Medication that is different from a prescriber's patient specific directions.

**15** Discrepancy between the prescriber's intended drug therapy and the drug therapy given to the patient.

**16** Error in the process of interpreting, verifying, and copying of medication orders.

**17** Mistake that occurs when the wrong medication is prescribed because of incorrect knowledge of the drug of choice.

**18** Error that has the potential to cause serious harm but did not do so in practice.

## FILL IN THE BLANKS

Fill in the blanks in each statement using the options in the box.
*Not all of them are required, so choose carefully!*

| | |
|---|---|
| avoidable | common |
| check | label |
| failure | strength |
| medication | multiple |
| costs | instructions |
| prescription | elderly |
| communication | selection |
| patient | quantity |

**19** A dispensing error can include the wrong drug for the patient, _____, formulation, _____ or incorrect _____ instructions.

**20** Poor _____ between primary and secondary care may result in the _____ to supply necessary medicines.

**21** Monitoring for side effects is important in _____ patients or people receiving _____ drug regimens.

**22** Slips, lapses, and failure to _____ actions can lead to a patient receiving the wrong _____, dose or _____ .

**23** Errors made when prescribing are the most _____ type of _____ medication error.

# ANSWERS

## TRUE OR FALSE?

**1** | **Drugs that are most commonly associated with medication errors have a wide therapeutic index.**

Drugs with a narrow therapeutic index are more likely to result in a medication error. A narrow index indicates that the blood concentration range between effective therapy and toxicity is small and therefore needs to be monitored closely.

**2** | **More prescribing errors are made by prescribers when they are unfamiliar with the drugs they are prescribing.**

Analysis of prescribing errors in hospitals found that prescribers made fewer errors when prescribing unfamiliar medicines. Errors were most likely to occur when prescribers were short of time and under pressure, making errors with drugs that they knew about and because they failed to check details for their specific patient.

**3** | **The majority of prescribing errors do not result in harm to the patient.**

The NPSA collects data on patient safety incidents. Medication incidents are the third largest group. Most medication errors are not harmful; however, a small proportion of these incidents will result in actual harm to patients. Many of these incidents are preventable.

**4** | **When writing a prescription, abbreviations should be avoided.**

Many abbreviations can be misinterpreted when transcribed or dispensed. Latin abbreviations should be avoided, as many of them are not understood by everyone. The abbreviations for the units of mass – micrograms and milligrams – can also be misunderstood. It is good practice to write out drug names and the units prescribed in full.

**5** | **Poor writing can lead to administration errors.**

Illegible handwriting can lead to errors in both the dispensing and administration of medications. The reader may misinterpret the drug name or misunderstand the dose to be given.

**6** | **Drug administration errors often result when one of the 'five cardinal rights' of drug administration are not followed.**

Administration errors can arise when the five cardinal rights are not followed correctly: right drug to the right patient, at the right dose, by the right route at the right time.

**7** It is usual when writing a drug dose to precede the
decimal point with a zero and to leave out trailing zeros.

The inappropriate use of decimal points can lead to large errors in a drug
dose. Zeros before a decimal point help to indicate that there is a decimal
point present (e.g. 0.25 mg); without the preceding zero this could be
read as 25 mg, a 100-fold increase in the dose. Trailing zeros, however,
could be misinterpreted, for instance 1.0 could be seen as a 10, also
leading to an overdose.

**8** Residents of care homes are particularly vulnerable to
medication errors.

Residents in care homes are particularly vulnerable because they might be
in more than one category of 'patients at most risk of a medication error'.
These include older adults (particularly the frail), multiple morbidities,
complex and hazardous medication regimens. They can have problems in
understanding or remembering to take medications and may have poor
compliance with their medications.

## a b c d MULTIPLE CHOICE

Correct answers identified in bold italics.

**9** Medication errors can be made by failing to check:

*a) for allergies to the medication*    b) for stocks in the pharmacy
c) directions on the packaging    d) the patient's date of birth

Errors in the choice of medication can occur when the practitioner
fails to find out enough information about the patient. They may then
prescribe a drug without realizing there is a contraindication, caution or
allergy. A full medical and medications history is necessary (this should
include questions about over-the-counter medicines, herbal remedies, and
recreational drugs) to ensure a prescribing error is avoided.

**10** Medication reviews ensure:

a) drug costs are reduced    b) contact with the patient is maintained
c) drug administration is correct    *d) side effects are detected*

Periodic medication reviews are important to ensure that side effects are
detected, laboratory tests are undertaken when necessary, patients are
given essential information about their medications, and participate in
decisions about their medicines.

**11** Communication problems with the patient can result in:

a) dispensing errors    b) fewer medicines to choose from
*c) incorrect use of medication*    d) improved safety of the patient

Communication problems can result in prescribing errors. Patients can suffer from adverse events because they do not understand their medical condition or how the drugs they are prescribed work and how the medication should be taken. They need to be given an appropriate explanation of their medication to avoid the incorrect usage.

**12** **When writing a prescription it is good practice:**

a) to use Latin abbreviations
b) to assume that a previous drug dose is correct
c) *to write units out in full*
d) to abbreviate drug names

Abbreviations should be avoided to reduce confusion between drug names that are similar. Latin abbreviations are considered acceptable but are not fully understood by everyone and so best practice would be to avoid their use. Because a drug dose was given before, it is not necessarily the case that the same dose is appropriate again; the previous dose might have been a loading dose. The treatment might not be working as expected. Writing drug dose units out in full can avoid confusion between micrograms and milligrams.

# MATCH THE TERMS

**13** Incorrect drug selection for the patient    **E.** prescribing error

**14** Medication that is different from a prescriber's patient specific directions.    **B.** dispensing error

**15** Discrepancy between the prescriber's intended drug therapy and the drug therapy given to the patient.    **A.** administration error

**16** Error in the process of interpreting, verifying, and copying of medication orders.    **F.** transcribing error

**17** Mistake that occurs when the wrong medication is prescribed because of incorrect knowledge of the drug of choice.    **C.** knowledge-related mistake

**18** Error that has the potential to cause serious harm but did not do so in practice.

**D. near miss**

## FILL IN THE BLANKS

**19** A dispensing error can include the wrong drug for the patient, *strength*, formulation, *quantity* or incorrect *label* instructions.

Dispensing errors are made at a pharmacy. They could be the result of poor handwriting on a prescription, an interruption during the dispensing process, or a misreading of drugs with a similar spelling.

**20** Poor *communication* between primary and secondary care may result in the *failure* to supply necessary medicines.

Good communication and record keeping are essential for safe prescribing. A lack of information, when patients are transferring between the different care systems, may also lead to inappropriate treatment as well as delays in essential medication.

**21** Monitoring for side effects is important in *elderly* patients or people receiving *multiple* drug regimens.

Older adults are more prone to side effects of drugs because they tend to be treated with several drugs for different conditions. Thus there is a greater likelihood of drugs interacting. In addition, older adults handle drugs differently to younger people because of altered pharmacokinetics (reduced drug metabolism and decreased excretion), leading to a greater potential for side effects to occur.

**22** Slips, lapses, and failure to *check* actions can lead to a patient receiving the wrong *prescription*, dose or *instructions*.

Pharmacists are an important checkpoint in the prescribing process. They can spot errors in doses and medications that interact. But failure to check allergy status during assessment will not be noticed. Checks are also important at the point of administration; failure to check a patient's identity can lead to a medicine being given to the wrong patient. Inappropriate or incorrect instructions could lead to ineffective therapy or poor concordance.

**23** Errors made when prescribing are the most *common* type of *avoidable* medication error.

Errors will always be made, as prescribers are human! It is important to reduce these errors and avoid their reoccurrence through good prescribing practice and processes.

# 11 Adverse drug reactions

## INTRODUCTION

When drugs are used clinically, there is always a risk that a person may react to a particular drug in a way that was not intended. Some of these reactions can be predicted with knowledge of the drug's pharmacology. Other reactions may not be predictable or even related to the dose of drug administered. Studies have found that approximately 4% of hospital admissions are due to adverse drug reactions and many of these are preventable (Pirmohamed et al., 2004; Howard et al., 2007). A small proportion of these reactions can be life threatening. Most drug reactions and drug–drug interactions are known and documented. It is therefore expected that prescribers will understand which groups of patients are most at risk and can reduce the risk of a patient having an adverse drug reaction, but also recognize these adverse reactions and deal with them appropriately.

---

**Useful resources**

Nurses Test Yourself in Pharmacology

---

**TRUE OR FALSE?**

Are the following statements true of false?

**1** Adverse drug reactions (ADRs) are more likely to occur in women.

**2** Tolerance to nicotine is an example of a chronic ADR.

**3** The toxic effect of drugs is always predictable.

**4** Disease progression can produce an ADR.

**5** ADRs are eliminated by careful clinical trials.

**6** Natural and herbal products do not cause ADRs.

**7** ADRs are more likely to occur when a drug has a narrow therapeutic window.

**8** Poor nutrition can result in an ADR.

**9** Drugs that are highly bound to plasma proteins will not interact when given in equal doses.

**10** All drug interactions will have a detrimental effect on the therapeutic outcomes of a patient.

**11** Drugs with a wide therapeutic window are less likely to induce an ADR.

**12** Nurse prescribers should not report ADRs.

**MULTIPLE CHOICE**

Identify one correct answer from each of the following.

**13** The adverse effects of drugs can be prevented by:

a) closely monitoring a patient's condition

b) changing the route of administration

c) changing the medication for an alternative drug

d) giving smaller doses of the drug more frequently

**14** Which of the following drugs is most likely to cause a drug reaction?

a) insulin

b) amoxycillin

c) salbutamol

d) warfarin

**15** A type 'A' adverse drug reaction:

a) is unpredictable and idiosyncratic

b) is produced by the long-term use of a drug

c) is dose dependent

d) occurs when a drug is stopped

**16** Which of the following patient groups is the most susceptible to ADRs?

a) Asians

b) older adults

c) males

d) the disabled

**17** The Yellow Card Scheme is a method of reporting:

   a) difficult patients

   b) suspected interactions of drugs

   c) medication errors

   d) drug compliance problems

**18** Which of the following actions will exacerbate an ADR?

   a) inform the patient

   b) increase the drug dose

   c) take only at night

   d) ignore the response

**19** In which of the following enzymes are genetic differences known to cause changes in the metabolism of drugs that can lead to ADRs?

   a) cyclooxygenase

   b) angiotensin converting enzyme

   c) cytochrome P450 enzymes

   d) acetylcholinesterase

**20** Which of the following commonly used drugs does not have a drug interaction with NSAIDs?

   a) enalapril

   b) lithium

   c) corticosteroids

   d) paracetamol

**21** Therapeutic drug monitoring of a drug's blood concentration is usually undertaken when a drug:

   a) has a narrow therapeutic window

b)  has a known drug interaction

c)  is very potent

d)  is known to cause side effects

**MATCH THE TERMS**

Identify which statement matches the description below.

- **A.** type A (augmented) drug reaction
- **B.** type B (bizarre) drug reaction
- **C.** serious adverse event
- **D.** delayed drug effect
- **E.** drug interaction
- **F.** side effect
- **G.** adverse drug reaction
- **H.** pharmacovigilance

**22** An expected and known effect of a drug that is not the intended therapeutic outcome.

**23** A dose-dependent effect that can be predicted from the drug's pharmacology.

**24** A harmful effect not predicted to occur within a drug's normal clinical dose range.

**25** An effect that occurs following a change in medication, food or drink.

**26** A reaction that becomes apparent months or years after exposure.

**27** The collection, monitoring, and evaluation of unexpected and unintended effects of medicines.

**28** Unpredictable response to a drug that is not related to drug dose.

**29** An untoward medical occurrence that is life-threatening, causes hospitalization or causes a persistent incapacity to the patient.

**FILL IN THE BLANKS**

Fill in the blanks in each statement using the options in the box.
*Not all of them are required, so choose carefully!*

| | |
|---|---|
| polypharmacy | common |
| side effects | wide |
| pharmacodynamic | bizarre |
| pharmacokinetics | interactions |
| rare | alternative |
| narrow | medications |
| hospitalization | concordance |
| toxicity | interactions |

**30** _____ is the term used when multiple _____ are used to treat many different disease states and can cause drug interactions and ADRs.

**31** Drug interactions can occur in any of the stages of _____.

**32** Drug reactions that have an unintended or harmful effect are _____ and can lead to _____.

**33** Complicated drug regimens risk creating drug _____ that may result in _____ problems with a patient's medications.

**34** When prescribing a new drug for a patient, the prescriber should always consider _____ with the patient's other drug treatments.

# ANSWERS

## TRUE OR FALSE?

**1** | Adverse drug reactions (ADRs) are more likely to occur in women.

Women are at greater risk of having an ADR than men. The reasons for this are not completely clear. It may be a result of hormonal differences as well as immunological factors. Pharmacokinetic factors may play a role. Women have a greater proportion of body fat than men, which may affect drug distribution. Drug doses tend to be 'one dose fits all', and women generally have a smaller body mass than men, which may predispose women towards a higher dose than men.

**2** | Tolerance to nicotine is an example of a chronic ADR.

Tolerance means that a drug dose that caused a particular response one day causes a reduced response to the drug after continued or chronic use. Thus a higher dose is required to get the same effect. The body reacts in an unintended way, making the drug less effective.

**3** | The toxic effect of drugs is always predictable.

Some adverse effects are predictable based on knowledge of their pharmacology (a type A ADR). Others are not predictable (a type B ADR).

**4** | Disease progression can produce an ADR.

Progression of a disorder to the gastrointestinal tract may alter the rate of absorption of the drug. Liver disease may reduce the metabolism of drugs and the composition of plasma proteins in the blood, thus affecting drug binding to these proteins. Kidney disease may reduce the elimination of drugs from the body. The above will tend to increase the drug levels within the body, increasing the likelihood of an ADR.

**5** | ADRs are eliminated by careful clinical trials.

Clinical trials carefully monitor the incidence of adverse effects that occur during a trial. However, a type B ADR is unpredictable and may occur in only a small percentage of patients and may not be picked up in a clinical trial.

**6** | Natural and herbal products do not cause ADRs.

Many herbal and natural products can cause ADRs. Many drugs have their origins as extracts from natural products. For instance, digoxin comes from the foxglove. St John's Wort, if taken in high doses, has many adverse effects and interacts with many drugs. Some foods can interact with drugs to cause ADRs.

**7** **ADRs are more likely to occur when a drug has a narrow therapeutic window.**

Drugs with a narrow therapeutic window have a limited range of concentrations in which they are effective. If they reach higher levels, they start to have toxic responses. Anything that interferes with these drugs to cause a rise in their concentration will increase the likelihood of an ADR.

**8** **Poor nutrition can result in an ADR.**

The metabolism of drugs relies on enzymes, many of which require co-factors derived from vitamins to function. The composition of plasma proteins is also dependent on dietary protein. If the diet is compromised, the functioning of these systems may also be compromised. Reduced drug metabolism will increase the drug levels in the body, which may lead to ADRs. A protein-poor diet will lead to a reduction of plasma proteins. Drugs that bind to these proteins will increase their free concentration leading to an increased risk of an ADR.

**9** **Drugs that are highly bound to plasma proteins will not interact when given in equal doses.**

Drugs that bind to plasma proteins will interact at any concentration. The consequences of these interactions depend on the ability of the drugs to bind to the proteins and the dose that is given. The more drug administered, the more likely a drug interaction will occur.

**10** **All drug interactions will have a detrimental effect on the therapeutic outcomes of a patient.**

Some drug interactions are beneficial to a patient if utilized properly, although many interactions are detrimental to the patient. Sinemet®, used in Parkinson's disease, is a combination of two drugs (carbidopa and L-dopa) that are used together deliberately to eliminate the side effects of L-dopa when used alone.

**11** **Drugs with a wide therapeutic window are less likely to induce an ADR.**

With a wide therapeutic window, a drug can be used over a larger range of doses with less likelihood of an unwanted response.

**12** **Nurse prescribers should not report ADRs.**

There is no restriction on who can report ADRs to the MHRA.

# MULTIPLE CHOICE

Correct answers are identified in bold italics.

**13** **The adverse effects of drugs can be prevented by:**

a) closely monitoring a patient's condition
b) changing the route of administration
*c) changing the medication for an alternative drug*
d) giving smaller doses of the drug more frequently

Stopping the medication causing the adverse effect altogether would be best, but the use of an alternative medication would still allow the treatment to continue.

**14** **Which of the following drugs is most likely to cause a drug reaction?**

a) insulin   b) amoxycillin   c) salbutamol   *d) warfarin*

Treatment with warfarin has to be monitored closely because it has a narrow therapeutic window. This means that the concentration of drug in the blood can easily reach toxic levels, causing an ADR.

**15** **A type 'A' adverse drug reaction:**

a) is unpredictable and idiosyncratic
b) is produced by the long-term use of a drug
*c) is dose dependent*
d) occurs when a drug is stopped

Type 'A' ADRs are predictable and dose dependent.

**16** **Which of the following patient groups is the most susceptible to ADRs?**

a) Asians   *b) older adults*   c) males   d) the disabled

Older adults have reduced liver and kidney function and are also the patient group that receives the majority of prescribed medicines.

**17** **The Yellow Card Scheme is a method of reporting:**

a) difficult patients   *b) suspected interactions of drugs*
c) medication errors   d) drug compliance problems

The Yellow Card Scheme is part of the MHRA. Reports can be made either by yellow cards found in the back of the BNF or online at yellowcard.mhra.gov.uk. It is an important means of gathering information on side effects and suspected interactions of medicines, vaccines, and complementary remedies. The information gathered from the scheme is continuously monitored to assess the risks to patients when taking medicines.

**18** **Which of the following actions will exacerbate an ADR?**

a) inform the patient    *b) increase the drug dose*

c) take only at night    d) ignore the response

If the response is a type A adverse drug reaction, it will be dose dependent. It would be best to stop the suspected drug, and if treatment is necessary, choose an alternative medicine.

**19** **In which of the following enzymes are genetic differences known to cause changes in the metabolism of drugs that can lead to ADRs?**

a) cyclooxygenase    b) angiotensin converting enzyme

*c) cytochrome P450 enzymes*    d) acetylcholinesterase

The cytochrome P450 family of enzymes is known to have genetic variations that affect the way drugs are metabolized. In some cases, this may mean that drugs are removed from the body faster, whereas other genetic variations may slow the removal of a drug.

**20** **Which of the following commonly used drugs does not have a drug interaction with NSAIDs?**

a) enalapril   b) lithium   c) corticosteroids   *d) paracetamol*

Appendix 1 of the BNF provides a list of most of the known drug–drug interactions. NSAIDs interact with many categories of drugs, but not paracetamol.

**21** **Therapeutic drug monitoring of a drug's blood levels is usually undertaken when a drug:**

*a) has a narrow therapeutic window*

b) has a known drug interaction

c) is very potent

d) is known to cause side effects

Therapeutic drug monitoring is carried out when the drug concentration in the blood needs to be maintained within a narrow therapeutic window. The dose needs to be kept at a level to achieve an optimal response to the drug with minimal toxicity to the patient.

**MATCH THE TERMS**

**22** An expected and known effect of a drug that is not the intended therapeutic outcome.

**F.** side effect

**23** A dose-dependent effect that can be predicted from the drug's pharmacology.

**A.** type A (augmented) drug reaction

**24** A harmful effect not predicted to occur within a drug's normal clinical dose range.

**G.** adverse drug reaction

**25** An effect that occurs following a change in medication, food or drink.

**E.** drug interaction

**26** A reaction that becomes apparent months or years after exposure.

**D.** delayed drug effect

**27** The collection, monitoring, and evaluation of unexpected and unintended effects of medicines.

**H.** pharmacovigilance

**28** Unpredictable response to a drug that is not related to drug dose.

**B.** type B (bizarre) drug reaction

**29** An untoward medical occurrence that is life-threatening, causes hospitalization or causes persistent incapacity to the patient.

**C.** serious adverse event

## FILL IN THE BLANKS

**30** *Polypharmacy* **is the term used when multiple** *medications* **are used to treat many different disease states and can cause drug interactions and ADRs.**

Polypharmacy is common in older adults when being treated for several co-morbidities. Multiple medications increase the possibility of an inter-action between the different drugs. It is important to monitor these patients for drug reactions that could adversely affect treatment, concordance or be life-threatening.

**31** **Drug interactions can occur in any of the stages of** *pharmacokinetics.*

Interactions at any of the four stages of pharmacokinetics can lead to increased or decreased effectiveness of a medicine. The dose may therefore need to be adjusted or an alternative medication prescribed.

**32** **Drug reactions that have an unintended or harmful effect are** *common* **and can lead to** *hospitalization.*

With drugs there is always a risk of an unwanted effect instead of the desired effect. Many drug reactions are known. Noxious drugs can require hospital treatment and may lead to the discontinuation of the drug.

**33** **Complicated drug regimens risk creating drug** *interactions* **that may result in** *concordance* **problems with a patient's medications.**

The more drugs taken by a patient, the greater the potential for drug interactions. If the dosing is complicated, requiring different drugs being taken at different times of the day, there is a greater the risk of drugs being taken at inappropriate times and this may result in an interaction. If these interactions cause unwanted symptoms or discomfort, then patients may not be taking medications appropriately, reducing concordance and the effectiveness of treatment.

**34** **When prescribing a new drug for a patient, the prescriber should always consider** *interactions* **with the patient's other drug treatments.**

It is best to avoid interactions in the first place. If these are considered at the start of treatment, the overall care will be more effective. If the prescriber does not consider interactions when prescribing, he or she will not have considered all the options and may be 'doing harm' as a result of an omission.

# 12 Cultural and religious issues

## INTRODUCTION

This chapter addresses cultural and religious awareness and looks at the influence of prescribers' attitudes on pharmaceutical decision making. Realizing that this decision making should be seen as a therapeutic alliance between the patient and the prescriber will help you to understand the factors that can influence the relationship and the factors that may have a significant impact on the outcome of treatment.

As healthcare professionals we are immersed in various cultures, which we belong to as part of our daily working and social lives. Culture reflects the whole of human behaviour, including values, attitudes, and ways of relating to and communicating with each other. Culture encompasses an individual's concept of self, universe, time, and space, as well as health, disease, and illness, and all of these may vary from those of our colleagues and indeed our patients. It therefore follows that our views may differ widely from those of our patients and this can have far-reaching implications in terms of safety, acceptability, and concordance.

Respect and good communication are essential components in the nurse–patient relationship and acknowledging a patient's personal beliefs and culture is an important part of the holistic approach to their care. Patients' beliefs may be fundamental to their health and well-being, and while many European cultures believe in the biomedical definition of illness and disease, other cultures have their own views. This may lead patients to ask for medicines or treatments that healthcare professionals do not feel are in the patients' best interests, or to refuse treatment which is in their best interests. We must not unfairly discriminate against patients by allowing personal views to adversely affect the relationship or the treatment we provide. What we need to try to do is balance nurses' and patients' conscience, religion, freedom of thought, and entitlement to care and treatment to meet clinical needs. We must also note the importance of discussing patients' beliefs, as we may sometimes wrongly ascribe certain beliefs or cultures to people simply based on stereotyping. The patient is the only person who knows how they wish to be treated, and whether we agree with them or not, respect is fundamental in understanding their wishes and achieving a positive outcome.

**Useful resources**

Leininger, M.M. and McFarland, M.R. (2002) *Transcultural Nursing: Concepts, Theories, Research and Practice.* New York: McGraw-Hill.

Cultural Diversity in Nursing
http://www.culturediversity.org/

**TRUE OR FALSE?**

Are the following statements true or false?

| 1 | In Chinese culture, iron is seen as a 'hot' medicine.

| 2 | Jehovah's Witnesses have strong objections to the use of blood and blood products, and may refuse them, even if there is a possibility that they may die as a result.

| 3 | All medication capsules contain animal-derived gelatine.

| 4 | It is not permissible for a person of the opposite sex to touch a Muslim patient.

| 5 | Breastfeeding mothers are not required to fast during Rosh Hashanah.

| 6 | Seventh Day Adventists adhere to kosher laws.

| 7 | Gelatine capsules are unsuitable for Buddhists.

| 8 | All drug companies mark medication packaging with ingredient labels and symbols.

| 9 | Pain relief in suppository form is permitted for Muslims during Ramadan.

| 10 | In Chinese culture, an excess of 'hot' foods such as chilli pepper, garlic, and onions is thought to cause stomach ache and diarrhoea.

**MULTIPLE CHOICE**

Identify one correct answer for each of the following.

**11** Stereotyping can be defined as:

a) a preconceived idea about another person or group of people, based on direct or indirect experiences

b) a fixed general image or set of characteristics that many people believe represent a particular type of person, group or thing

c) the term used for categorizing a person or group of people, based on another's experience

d) a negative response to a person from a particular group

**12** Prejudice can be defined as:

a) a preconceived opinion that is not based on reason or actual experience

b) the tendency to dislike people because of their characteristics or culture

c) a negative behavioural tendency with respect to the persons who are the object of prejudice

d) behaviour directed towards individuals on the basis of their membership of a particular group

**13** In Asian philosophy, the concept of Yin and Yang represents:

a) good and evil

b) polar opposites

c) hot and cold forces that counteract each other and negate the existence of the other in order to allow balance in the natural world

d) all of the above

**14** Why are people with diabetes sometimes exempt from some celebrations of the Jewish festival Rosh Hashanah?

a) because it involves foods with a very high sugar content

b) because they are expected to fast and this would be dangerous

c) because they are not allowed to use porcine insulin during the festival

d) because the use of injectable medication is forbidden

**15** The study of a culture is termed:

a) sociology

b) anthropology

c) culturology

d) ethnography

**16** In Chinese culture, which of the following foods would be seen as a 'cold' food?

a) mango

b) turkey

c) orange

d) beef

**17** Who are *not* exempt from fasting during Ramadan?

a) pregnant women

b) breastfeeding mothers

c) adolescents

d) those travelling

**18** The best person to translate for a patient whose first language is not English is:

a) the person who accompanies them

b) a son or daughter who knows them well

c)  a translator

d)  a healthcare professional who speaks their language


**19**  The Sabbath is the most important of Jewish Holy Days. It starts:

a)  at sunset on Friday and lasts until sunset on Saturday evening

b)  at sunset on Saturday and lasts until sunset on Sunday evening

c)  at sunrise on Sunday and lasts until sunset

d)  at sunrise on Saturday and lasts until sunset


**20**  Sikhs are not permitted:

a)  to bathe in running water

b)  to cut any body hair

c)  to eat fish

d)  to hold hands in public

## MATCH THE TERMS

Match each term with the correct description.

- **A.** ethnicity
- **B.** culture
- **C.** ethnocentrism
- **D.** empowerment
- **E.** acculturation
- **F.** kosher
- **G.** halal

**21** Ritually fit or allowed to be eaten or used, according to dietary or ceremonial laws.

**22** The perception that one's own way of viewing the world is best.

**23** Cultural patterns linked to nationalities or countries.

**24** A complex pattern of shared meanings, beliefs, and behaviours that are learned and acquired by a group of people during the course of history.

**25** Meat from animals that have been killed according to Muslim law.

**26** The level to which a person adopts the traits of a new culture.

**27** The process by which people gain greater control over decisions and actions that affect their health.

## FILL IN THE BLANKS

Fill in the blanks in each statement using the options in the box.

*Not all of them are required, so choose carefully!*

| | |
|---|---|
| touch | Lights |
| Jewish | Hindu |
| non-verbal | Sign |
| Ramadan | Muslim |
| water | deaf |
| Buddhist | hearing |

**28** Hanukkah or Chanukkah is the _____ Festival of _____.

**29** Haptics refers to the sense of _____ _____ and is a form of _____ communication.

**30** Karma is a principle in both the _____ and _____ religions.

**31** Eid is a _____ holiday that marks the end of _____, the Islamic holy month of fasting (sawm).

**32** A language that makes use of space and involves movement of the hands, body, face, and head is known as British _____ Language and is a way that _____ people communicate.

## LABELLING EXERCISE

Which religions do the symbols in the box relate to?

| | |
|---|---|
| Seventh Day Adventist | Judaism |
| Hindu | Christianity |
| Buddhism | Sikh |

**Figure 12.1**

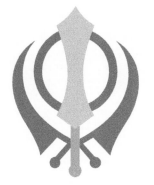

33 _____

34 _____

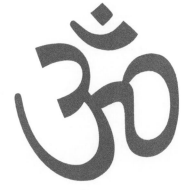

35 _____

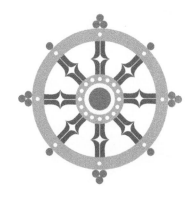

36 _____

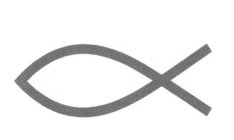 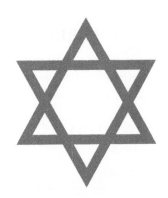

**37** _____      **38** _____

# ANSWERS

## TRUE OR FALSE?

**1** **In Chinese culture, iron is seen as a 'hot' medicine.**

Chinese culture often categorizes conditions and treatments as either 'hot' or 'cold'. To treat a 'hot' condition you need to use a 'cold' remedy to help restore balance and health. Pregnancy is seen as a 'hot' condition and iron tablets are seen as a 'hot' remedy, thus difficulties may arise when trying to treat a pregnant woman with anaemia.

**2** **Jehovah's Witnesses have strong objections to the use of blood and blood products, and may refuse them, even if there is a possibility that they may die as a result.**

Accepting a blood transfusion willingly and without regret is seen as a sin. The Witness concerned would no longer be regarded as one of Jehovah's Witnesses. This often includes autologous transfusions, although some Witnesses will accept this.

**3** **All medication capsules contain animal derived-gelatine.**

Capsules are made from aqueous solutions of gelling agents that can include animal protein (mainly gelatine) but also plant polysaccharides or their derivatives, such as carrageenans and modified forms of starch and cellulose.

**4** **It is not permissible for a person of the opposite sex to touch a Muslim patient.**

Modesty is crucial to Muslims and they are often offended and shocked by nakedness. Where possible, Muslim women should always be examined by female doctors and nurses and Muslim men by male doctors and nurses.

**5** **Breastfeeding mothers are not required to fast during Rosh Hashanah.**

During Rosh Hashanah, males and females over the age of Bar and Bat Mitzvah respectively fast from dawn until nightfall (in commemoration of the assassination of Gedaliah, governor of Judea). However, pregnant and nursing mothers do not have to observe the fast and those who are ill will usually consult their Rabbi.

**6**   **Seventh Day Adventists adhere to kosher laws.**

Adventists are known for presenting a 'health message' that recommends vegetarianism and expects adherence to the kosher laws in Leviticus 11. Obedience to these laws means abstinence from pork, shellfish, and other foods proscribed as 'unclean'.

**7**   **Gelatine capsules are unsuitable for Buddhists.**

Not all Buddhists are vegetarians. The early Buddhist monastic code banned monks from eating meat if the animal had been killed specifically to feed them, but otherwise instructed them to eat anything they were given. As nurse prescribers we should be aware of patients' beliefs and remember that people do not always realize what is in the medications they are taking. The same applies to vegetarians and vegans. Thus joint decision making helps to ensure that we respect all patients' needs and beliefs.

**8**   **All drug companies mark medication packaging with ingredient labels and symbols.**

This is not a legal requirement. In 1992, the European Commission issued a Directive on the labelling of medicinal products for human use and on package leaflets. The legislation requires that the patient information leaflet contained within drug packaging should be drawn up in accordance with the Summary of Product Characteristics and should contain specific pieces of information in a specific order. Medication packaging itself is not required to display this and if nurses/patients wish to find out about specific ingredients in their medications, they would need to speak to a pharmacist or the manufacturer of the drug.

**9**   **Pain relief in suppository form is permitted for Muslims during Ramadan.**

While fasting, Muslims do not take anything into their body by mouth, nose, injection or suppository from dawn to sunset. This can make the provision of pain relief difficult, but it must be borne in mind that participating in the fast will give great comfort to the patient. Taking advice from the Imam may be helpful (although generally speaking the Imam is the leader of ritual prayer in the mosque, many also take on pastoral roles).

**10**   **In Chinese culture, an excess of 'hot' foods such as chilli pepper, garlic, and onions is thought to cause stomach ache and diarrhoea.**

Some foods that belong to the Yang (also known as 'hot' food) are chilli pepper, garlic, onion, curry, cabbage, eggplant, pineapple, cherry, peanuts, shrimp, crab, French fries, fried chicken, and pizza. Excessive intake of these foods is thought to cause skin rashes, hives, pimples, nose bleeds, bloating, indigestion, constipation, redness in the eyes, and sore throat. In contrast, an excess of 'cold' (Yin) foods is thought to cause diarrhoea, stomach ache, dizziness, and weakness.

**MULTIPLE CHOICE**

Correct answers identified in bold italics.

**11** **Stereotyping can be defined as:**

a) a preconceived idea about another person or group of people, based on direct or indirect experiences

b) *a fixed general image or set of characteristics that many people believe represent a particular type of person, group or thing*

c) the term used for categorizing a person or group of people, based on another's experience

d) a negative response to a person from a particular group

**12** **Prejudice can be defined as:**

a) *a preconceived opinion that is not based on reason or actual experience*

b) the tendency to dislike people because of their characteristics or culture

c) a negative behavioural tendency with respect to the persons who are the object of prejudice

d) behaviour directed towards individuals on the basis of their membership of a particular group

**13** **In Asian philosophy, the concept of Yin and Yang represents:**

a) good and evil

b) *polar opposites, or seemingly contrary forces, that are interconnected and interdependent in the natural world*

c) hot and cold forces that counteract each other and negate the existence of the other in order to allow balance in the natural world

d) all of the above.

**14** **Why are people with diabetes sometimes exempt from some celebrations of the Jewish festival Rosh Hashanah?**

a) *because it involves foods with a very high sugar content*

b) because they are expected to fast and this would be dangerous

c) because they are not allowed to use porcine insulin during the festival

d) because the use of injectable medication is forbidden.

Rosh Hashanah is the Jewish New Year festival that lasts two days. A lot of time is spent in the synagogue during Rosh Hashanah and afterwards special foods such as apples dipped in honey and sweet carrot stew are eaten as a symbol of the sweet New Year that each Jew hopes lies ahead.

**15** **The study of a culture is termed:**

a) sociology  b) anthropology  c) culturology  *d) ethnography*

Ethnography is a qualitative research method for learning and understanding cultural phenomena that reflect the knowledge and system of meanings guiding the life of a cultural group. Anthropology is the study of human origin, behaviour, and development. Culturology is a branch of anthropology concerned with the study of cultural institutions as distinct from the people who are involved in them. Sociology is the study of human society.

**16** **In Chinese culture, which of the following foods would be seen as a 'cold' food?**

a) mango  b) turkey  *c) orange*  d) beef

Foods belonging to the Yin (also known as 'cold' foods) are bitter melon, winter melon, Chinese greens, mustard greens, watercress, Napa cabbage, bean sprout, soybean, mung bean, tulip, water chestnut, cilantro, orange, watermelon, banana, coconut, cucumber, beer, pop, ice cream, ice chips, grass jelly, clams, and oysters.

**17** **Who is *not* exempt from fasting during Ramadan?**

a) pregnant women  b) breastfeeding mothers  *c) adolescents*

d) those travelling

It is compulsory for all Muslims over the age of 12 to fast during Ramadan. Fasting is the duty of every adult Muslim, but there are some exceptions. Older adults, sick, pregnant women, nursing mothers, and travellers do not have to fast but they must fast at a convenient time later on. The fast begins at dawn and ends at sunset, throughout the month of Ramadan. During this time, eating, drinking, smoking, and having sex are strictly forbidden.

**18** **The best person to translate for a patient whose first language is not English is:**

a)  the person who accompanies them

b)  a son or daughter who knows them well

*c)  a translator*

d)  a healthcare professional who speaks their language

It is always best practice to use a translator for such consultations. Children and other family members may misinterpret what is being said by either the nurse or the patient, or may be embarrassed if the issues are sensitive. Using another healthcare professional may have benefits with regards to understanding terminology but patients may not be happy with this if they know the individual, or it may be that there is bias or an assumption that does not reflect the true consultation. A qualified translator will ensure that questions are asked as you speak them. Make sure you still direct your questions to the patient and that the patient knows the consultation will be confidential.

**19** **The Sabbath is the most important of Jewish Holy Days. It starts:**

a) *at sunset on Friday and lasts until sunset on Saturday evening*

b) at sunset on Saturday and lasts until sunset on Sunday evening

c) at sunrise on Sunday and lasts until sunset

d) at sunrise on Saturday and lasts until sunset

The Sabbath is a time when families come together in the presence of God in their own homes. All chores and work must be completed before sunset on Friday. It is a day of rest and giving thanks.

**20** **Sikhs are not permitted:**

a) to bathe in running water    *b) to cut any body hair*

c) to eat fish    d) to hold hands in public

Sikhs believe many things about body hair, including that hair is a gift from God and should be kept as God created it. They also believe that they should bow their head only to the Guru, not a barber, and that not cutting the hair is a symbol of moving beyond the concerns of the body. This may have implications when prescribing medications that come in patch form or when shaving is required to insert a cannula, etc. This applies to both men and women.

 **MATCH THE TERMS**

**21** Ritually fit or allowed to be eaten or used, according to the dietary or ceremonial laws.   **F.** kosher

**22** The perception that one's own way of viewing the world is best.   **C.** ethnocentrism

**23** Cultural patterns linked to nationalities or countries.   **A.** ethnicity

**24** A complex pattern of shared meanings, beliefs, and behaviours that are learned and acquired by a group of people during the course of history.   **B.** culture

**25** Meat from animals that have been killed according to Muslim law.

**G.** halal

**26** The level to which a person adopts the traits of a new culture.

**E.** acculturation

**27** The process through which people gain greater control over decisions and actions that affect their health.

**D.** empowerment

## FILL IN THE BLANKS

**28** **Hanukkah or Chanukkah is the _Jewish_ Festival of _Lights_.**

The festival dates back to two centuries before the start of Christianity. In the western calendar, Hanukkah is celebrated in November or December using lighted candles (eight candles – one each day) symbolizing how God took care of His people.

**29** **Haptics refers to the sense of _touch_ and is a form of _non-verbal_ communication.**

Touching is treated differently from one country to another and socially acceptable levels of touching vary from one culture to another. For example, in Western Europe people are less likely to touch during communication whereas Eastern Europeans use touch more frequently. Touching the head in Thai culture is seen as very disrespectful.

**30** **Karma is a principle in both the _Hindu_ and _Buddhist_ religions.**

Karma is defined as the total effect of a person's actions and conduct during the successive phases of the person's existence, regarded as determining the person's destiny.

**31** **Eid is a _Muslim_ holiday that marks the end of _Ramadan_, the Islamic holy month of fasting (sawm).**

Eid is an Arabic word meaning 'festivity'. The holiday celebrates the conclusion of the 29 or 30 days of dawn-to-sunset fasting during the entire month of Ramadan.

**32** A language that makes use of space and involves movement of the hands, body, face, and head is known as British *Sign* Language and is a way that *deaf* people communicate.

British Sign Language (BSL) is the sign language used in the United Kingdom, and is the first or preferred language of some deaf people in the UK. More than 125,000 deaf adults in the UK use BSL, as well as an estimated 20,000 children.

 **LABELLING EXERCISE**

Which religions do the symbols relate to?

**Figure 12.2**

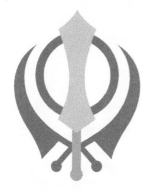 

**33** Sikh

**34** Seventh Day Adventist

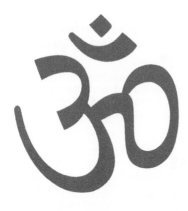

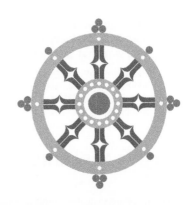

**35** Hindu

**36** Buddhism

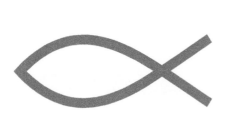

**37** Christianity

**38** Judaism

# 13 Concordance

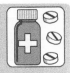

## INTRODUCTION

Prescribed medicines are the most common form of medical intervention and account for approximately £8.2 billion of NHS expenditure each year, and yet it has been estimated that about half of those for whom medicines are prescribed do not take them in the recommended way. Until recently, this was termed non-compliance; sometimes seen as a manifestation of irrational behaviour or wilful failure to observe instructions. However, forgetfulness is among the more common reasons for not taking medications as directed, and we now prefer to talk about concordance, adherence or non-adherence to a regimen.

As nurse prescribers we have the ability to make a difference to patients, the Health Service, and society in general simply by making sure that we are aware of the reasons behind non-concordance and the impact it has. Non-concordance has huge economic and personal consequences and results in ill-health, approximately 10% of all hospitalizations each year, and can even result in death. It reduces quality of life, increases waste, and is an unnecessary cost to the economy. However, non-concordance can often be dealt with easily and effectively.

In many cases, non-concordance can be seen as a fundamental weakness in the delivery of health care, often because of failure by clinicians to fully agree treatment with the patient, or as a result of lack of support following diagnosis and management of their condition. Understanding patients' perspectives of medicines and the reasons why they may not want or are unable to use them can help to address issues of non-concordance, and healthcare professionals have a duty to help patients make informed decisions about treatment and using prescribed medications appropriately.

> Increasing the effectiveness of adherence interventions may have a far greater impact on the health of the population than any improvement in specific medical treatments. (Haynes, 2001, cited in WHO, 2003)

## Useful resources

NICE (2009) *Medicines Adherence: Involving Patients in Decisions about Prescribed Medicines and Supporting Adherence* (CG76). London: NICE.

World Health Organization (2003) *Adherence to Long-term Therapies: Evidence for Action*. Geneva: WHO. Available at: http://apps.who.int/medicinedocs/en/d/Js4883e/5.html.

## TRUE OR FALSE?

Are the following statements true or false?

**1** Patients on regular medication for chronic diseases are most likely to have the best rates of concordance.

**2** Most non-concordance is intentional.

**3** Giving more information improves concordance.

**4** Students of Asian cultural background are more likely to perceive medicines as intrinsically harmful.

**5** There is strong evidence to suggest that self-management programmes offered to patients with chronic diseases improve health status and reduce utilization and costs.

**6** Non-concordance is not consistently related to age, gender, social class, education, personality or type of disease.

**7** Reducing the frequency of drug administration improves concordance.

**8** Hypertensive patients have high rates of non-concordance.

**9** Non-concordance issues are most frequent in patients with short-term conditions.

To help patients remember medications and what they have been prescribed for, it is acceptable to write a description of the action of the drug on a prescription, for example, 'sleeping tablet' on a zopiclone prescription.

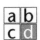 **MULTIPLE CHOICE**

Identify one correct answer for each of the following.

**11** A patient's recall of information given to them by a clinician is *least* likely to be affected by:

a) the patient's intellectual level

b) the importance of the information to the patient

c) the time of day the information is given

d) repetition of information

**12** The key reason for patients' non-concordance to ipratropium aerosol inhalation is:

a) palpitations

b) inability to use device appropriately

c) difficult dosing regime

d) dry mouth

**13** Which of the following is *least* likely to aid concordance?

a) patient information leaflet in medication packaging

b) dosette boxes

c) simplifying dose regimen

d) patient-centred consultations

**14** A common reason given by patients for stopping taking ACE inhibitors is:

a) diarrhoea

b) constipation

c) cough

d) dry mouth

**15** What percentage of patients with asthma take their medications as prescribed?

   a) 20%
   b) 30%
   c) 40%
   d) 50%

**16** Which of the following factors is related to intentional non-concordance?

   a) swallowing difficulties
   b) cognitive issues
   c) patient's health beliefs
   d) incorrect medication prescribed

**17** Leventhal's self-regulation theory (Leventhal et al., 1980) is essentially based around:

   a) the patient's capacity to improve their health
   b) the patient's willingness to improve their health
   c) the clinician's ability to guide the patient
   d) the clinician's ability to control a consultation

**18** Weinstein (1983) noted that in general people believe they are less likely to suffer from health problems than other people of the same age and sex and that certain factors contribute to this unrealistic optimism. Which of the following does *not* contribute?

   a) the belief that if it hasn't happened yet, it won't
   b) the belief that problems are infrequent
   c) personal experience of a problem
   d) problems are preventable by individuals

**19** Which of the following is *not* a motivating factor for patients to take medication?

a) when they understand and accept their diagnosis

b) when they agree with the treatment proposed

c) when they have their concerns about the medicines addressed specifically

d) when they understand the side effects of the medication

**20** Approximately what percentage of patients leave the consultation room unclear of what they have been told?

a) 30%

b) 40%

c) 50%

d) 60%

**MATCH THE TERMS**

Match each term with the correct description:

    **A.** unintentional non-concordance

    **B.** compliance

    **C.** primacy effect

    **D.** patient information leaflet (PIL)

    **E.** intentional non-concordance

    **F.** adherence

    **G.** patient-centred

**21** Relating to beliefs and concerns or problems about medicines.

**22** It is a legal requirement that this information is included within the packaging of a medication.

**23** Relating to practical problems such as inappropriate formulation of medicines.

**24** The extent to which a person's behaviour corresponds with agreed recommendations from a healthcare provider.

**25** Recalling information told first better than later information.

**26** Respecting and responsive to individual patient preferences and needs.

**27** Willingness to follow a prescribed course of treatment.

# FILL IN THE BLANKS

Fill in the blanks in each statement using the options in the box.

*Not all of them are required, so choose carefully!*

| | |
|---|---|
| 50 | multidisciplinary |
| hospitalization | threat |
| patient-centred | 70 |
| illness | empowerment |
| behaviour | health |
| deaths | 20 |

**28** Leventhal's self-regulation theory postulates that _____ representa-tions determine a person's appraisal of an illness situation and their subsequent _____ behaviour.

**29** The Health Belief Model suggests that your belief in a personal _____ together with your belief in the effectiveness of the proposed _____ will predict the likelihood of that behaviour occurring.

**30** Concordance sufficient to attain therapeutic objectives occurs approxi-mately ___% of the time with one in six patients taking medication exactly as directed and ___% of prescriptions never cashed.

**31** Approximately ___% of patients want to be more involved in decisions about their treatment. Joint decision making has been shown to aid _____ of patients and improve concordance.

**32** Non-concordance is thought to contribute to between 18% and 48% of asthma _____. It also leads to increased _____ and non-medical costs, which contribute to a decreased quality of life.

**33** Concordance can be aided by a _____ _____ approach using _____ care.

# ANSWERS

## TRUE OR FALSE?

**1** | **Patients on regular medication for chronic diseases are most likely to have the best rates of concordance.**

Research shows that up to 50% of patients with long-term conditions have problems with concordance. This may be related to polypharmacy, age or difficulty understanding difficult dosing regimes, but also the fact that many long-term conditions are self-managed and require appropriate decision making and consultation at the beginning to ensure regimes are followed.

**2** | **Most non-concordance is intentional.**

Intentional non-concordance results from conscious decisions by the patient about a multitude of things, including illness, medications, experience, culture, lifestyle, religion, and education. All of these will influence a decision to take or not take a medication. However, this should not lead to patient blame. There continues to be a tendency to focus on patient-related factors as the causes of problems with concordance, when it has been shown that factors that make up the healthcare environment in which patients receive care have a marked effect on concordance. Patients may also become frustrated if their preferences in treatment-related decisions are not taken into account, and studies have shown that patients who feel less empowered in relation to treatment decisions have more negative attitudes towards their treatment.

**3** | **Giving more information improves concordance.**

This isn't always the case. If we bombard patients with information or give it to them in ways they do not understand, they will not be able to make an informed judgement about whether to take the medication or not. Also, if we do not provide the information that is important to them, they will not be satisfied and thus less likely to take a drug. It is important to understand the patient's perspective on their illness and how it could/should be treated.

**4** | **Students of Asian cultural background are more likely to perceive medicines as intrinsically harmful.**

A survey of undergraduate students in the UK of Asian and European cultural backgrounds identified differences between groups in beliefs about medicines (modern pharmaceuticals) and personal sensitivity to the adverse effects of taking medicines (Horne et al., 2004). Students of Asian cultural background were significantly more likely to perceive medicines as intrinsically harmful, addictive substances that should be avoided and less likely to endorse the benefits of modern medicines.

**5** **There is strong evidence to suggest that self-management programmes offered to patients with chronic diseases improve health status and reduce utilization and costs.**

Self-management and concordance programmes, combined with regular treatment and disease-specific education, produce significant improvements in health-promoting behaviours, cognitive symptom management, communication, and disability management. It has also been demonstrated that such programmes appear to result in a reduction in the numbers of patients being hospitalized, days in hospital, and outpatient visits.

**6** **Non-concordance is not consistently related to age, gender, social class, education, personality or type of disease.**

Most people are non-adherent some of the time.

**7** **Reducing the frequency of drug administration improves concordance.**

Although it makes sense to reduce the administration of drugs to once or at most twice a day, there is little evidence to suggest it aids concordance. Taking the time to explain the benefits and adverse effects of a drug are more important in aiding concordance than whether the patient has to take the medication once or four times a day.

**8** **Hypertensive patients have high rates of non-concordance.**

This is often due to multiple treatment regimes, side effects of drugs, and the fact that most hypertensive patients experience few/no symptoms before they are diagnosed. The new guidelines of the British Hypertension Society (NICE, 2011) have simplified treatment of hypertension but many patients are still on old regimes that involve three or more drugs. However, if this regime is working for the patient, then it may be wise to leave well alone.

**9** **Non-concordance issues are more frequent in patients with short-term conditions.**

There is much greater concordance if a disease or illness is short term, symptomatic, painful, and publicly distressing. Patients with visible skin conditions or sexually transmitted infections tend to be more concordant in general. Much lower concordance rates are found in patients with long-term conditions due to a number of factors, including complicated medication regimens, whether medication was used to cure or prevent, and how medications impact lifestyle.

| 10 | **To help patients remember medications and what they have been prescribed for, it is acceptable to write a description of the action of the drug on a prescription, for example, 'sleeping tablet' on a zopiclone prescription.** |

It is perfectly acceptable to write information like this on a prescription, but it must be written in inverted commas. All other information as outlined in the British National Formulary (BNF) on the writing of prescriptions *must* also be on the prescription but often this description will help patients on multiple regimes to remember which medicine does what and may also therefore aid concordance.

 **MULTIPLE CHOICE**

Correct answers identified in bold italics.

| 11 | **A patient's recall of information given to them by a clinician is *least* likely to be affected by:** |

a) the patient's intellectual level

b) the importance of the information to the patient

*c) the time of day the information is given*

d) repetition of information

There is little evidence to suggest that our recall of information is affected by time of day, particularly when you bear in mind the varied daily routines of people. However, we do know that the other three factors will impact recall significantly, along with primacy, simplicity, and specificity of the information given.

| 12 | **The key reason for patients' non-concordance to ipratropium aerosol inhalation is:** |

a) palpitations    *b) inability to use device appropriately*

c) difficult dosing regime    d) dry mouth

Poor education of how to use an inhaler device is still the most common reason for lack of concordance to inhalers in general. Palpitations are a rare side effect of antimuscarinic bronchodilators and although dosin is usually 3–4 times daily, this dosing regime is less likely to affe concordance than an inability to use the device. Dry mouth is the m common side effect of the medication, but again this is generally dov poor inhaler technique.

| 13 | **Which of the following is *least* likely to aid concordance?** |

*a) patient information leaflet in medication packaging*

b) dosette boxes

c)  simplifying dose regimen

d)  patient-centred consultations

A statutory framework across the European Union requires the provision of a statutory patient information leaflet (PIL) with every medicine supplied to a patient at any time. These leaflets describe in detail what the medicine is for, its dose, interactions with food and other medicines, and possible side effects. While this may be viewed as useful, it has also been seen to be problematic. Not only are the leaflets densely typed and difficult to read, but often patients and their carers are concerned about potential side effects and research has suggested that patients believe the information to be of little value to them.

**14 A common reason given by patients for stopping taking ACE inhibitors is:**

a) diarrhoea  b) constipation  *c) cough*  d) dry mouth

ACE inhibitors regularly cause dry cough, which may be very troublesome to patients, although generally it is more troublesome to their families. Educating patients that they may experience a dry cough and ways of managing it can be extremely useful in aiding understanding and therefore concordance to these drugs. However, often a change in anti-hypertensive to an angiotensin receptor blocker (ARB) is required and patients should be advised that there are other options should their side effects prove troublesome to their daily life.

**15 What percentage of patients with asthma take their medications as prescribed?**

*a) 20%*  b) 30%  c) 40%  d) 50%

Approximately 80% of patients with asthma do not adhere to medication regimes. This may be due to age, poor understanding of their disease, or an inability to use inhaler devices appropriately.

**16 Which of the following factors is related to intentional non-concordance?**

a) swallowing difficulties  b) cognitive issues
*c) patient's health beliefs*  d) incorrect medication prescribed

What a patient believes about their illness and the medication prescribed to treat it will have a huge impact on whether they adhere to a certain regime. For example, if they perceive the risks of treatment to outweigh the risk of the illness, they are less likely to take the medication. Patients may also be concerned about perceived side effects of medication or becoming dependent on certain drugs. As nurse prescribers we need to ensure that we identify patients' beliefs and concerns so that these issues can be resolved and the patient can be involved in the decision-making process.

**17** **Leventhal's self-regulation theory (Leventhal et al., 1980) is essentially based around:**

a) the patient's capacity to improve their health

*b) the patient's willingness to improve their health*

c) the clinician's ability to guide the patient

d) the clinician's ability to control a consultation.

Self-regulation theory is a system of conscious personal health management. Although a clinician may give a patient sound advice, the theory states that only with self-regulation will the patient use that advice appropriately. For medical treatment to be effective, the patient must want to improve their health.

**18** **Weinstein (1983) noted that in general people believe they are less likely to suffer from health problems than other people of the same age and sex and that certain factors contribute to this unrealistic optimism. Which of the following does *not* contribute?**

a) the belief that if it hasn't happened yet, it won't

b) the belief that problems are infrequent

*c) personal experience of a problem*

d) problems are preventable by individuals

If a person has personal experience of a problem, they are more likely to believe that certain health problems could happen to them in the future. Unrealistic optimism is fuelled by people believing that if it hasn't already happened then it won't, that health problems are less frequent than we are led to believe, and that they are able to prevent health problems and therefore it won't happen to them. People show 'selective focus' and have unrealistic ideas about their chances of experiencing health problems.

**19** **Which of the following is *not* a motivating factor for patients to take medication?**

a) when they understand and accept their diagnosis

b) when they agree with the treatment proposed

c) when they have their concerns about the medicines addressed specificall

*d) when they understand the side effects of the medicine*

Although understanding side effects of medicines is important to help concordance, this is not a key motivator for patients to actually take medication; indeed, it may have an adverse effect on motivation if r are worried about unpleasant side effects. Patients' beliefs about all illness, their medication, and the perceived risks versus benefits important for motivating them to follow a specific drug regime.

**20** **Approximately what percentage of patients leave the consultation room unclear of what they have been told?**

a) 30%   b) 40%   c) 50%   d) 60%

Patient communication encompasses interventions ranging from physician–patient communication, sending mail or telephonic reminders, to involving patients' families in the dialogue. Of these, the most problematic is physician–patient communication. At least 50% of patients leave their doctors' offices not knowing what they have been told (Atreja et al., 2005).

 ## MATCH THE TERMS

**21** Relating to beliefs and concerns or problems about medicines.

E. intentional non-concordance

**22** It is a legal requirement that this information is included within the packaging of a medication.

D. patient information leaflet (PIL)

**23** Relating to practical problems such as inappropriate formulation of medicines.

A. unintentional non-concordance

**24** The extent to which a person's behaviour corresponds with agreed recommendations from a healthcare provider.

F. adherence

Recalling information told first better than later information.

C. primary effect

Respecting and responsive to individual patient preferences and needs.

G. patient-centred

**27** Willingness to follow a prescribed course of treatment.

B. compliance

# FILL IN THE BLANKS

**28** Leventhal's self-regulation theory postulates that *illness* representations determine a person's appraisal of an illness situation and their subsequent *health* behaviour.

This relates to how serious we view an illness and how likely we believe we are to suffer from that illness. Thus if we see an illness as minor, we are less likely to engage in behaviour to prevent it. Similarly, if we feel we are unlikely to develop a certain illness, this prevents us engaging in positive health behaviour or stopping negative health behaviour.

**29** The Health Belief Model suggests that your belief in a personal *threat* together with your belief in the effectiveness of the proposed *behaviour* will predict the likelihood of that behaviour occurring.

If you believe that you are unlikely to become more unwell from a certain condition and if you also believe that management of that condition is unlikely to be effective, then you are less likely to follow advice on the management of that condition.

**30** Concordance sufficient to attain therapeutic objectives occurs approximately *50*% of the time with one in six patients taking medication exactly as directed and *20%* of prescriptions never cashed.

This is often linked to poor education and the patient not being included in the consultation process. Patient-centred care has been found time and again to improve outcomes, particularly through improved concordance.

**31** Approximately *70%* of patients want to be more involved in decisions about their treatment. Joint decision making has been shown to aid *empowerment* of patients and improve concordance.

When we ensure that patients are involved in their care they are more likely to accept and therefore adhere to management regimes.

**32** Non-concordance is thought to contribute to between 18% and 48% of asthma *deaths*. It also leads to increased *hospitalization* and non-medical costs, which contribute to a decreased quality of life.

Many of the issues surrounding non-concordance are linked to poor education about asthma, its symptoms, management, and severity.

**33** **Concordance can be aided by a _multidisciplinary_ approach using _patient-centred_ care.**

This ensures that the members of the multidisciplinary team and the patient himself or herself are partners in the care and management of the patient, and that they fully understand the management and are cognisant of any changes and the impact these may have.

# Glossary

**Absorption:** in pharmacology, the passage of drugs from the administration site into the body.

**Accountability:** healthcare professionals are responsible to their patients, their employers, their professional body, and the law for their actions and omissions while undertaking their job.

**Adverse reaction:** a noxious or unintended reaction to an administered drug.

**Blood–brain barrier:** a physical barrier that prevents potentially harmful chemicals in the blood passing into the brain, while allowing nutrients to cross.

**Borderline substance:** in some circumstances, foods have the properties of drugs (e.g. enteral feeds or nutritional supplements).

**Cautionary labels:** also called cautionary and advisory labels, they offer advice on how medications should be taken, stored, with warnings or any side effects that might be anticipated when taking the medicines to ensure the effectiveness of the treatment.

**Clearance:** the elimination of a drug from the body.

**Conjugation:** in drug metabolism, the joining of two chemicals together.

**Contra-indication:** a condition or factor that makes a treatment inadvisable.

**Controlled drug:** a potentially harmful and addictive drug, the manufacture, supply, and possession of which is restricted by the Misuse of Drugs Act 1971.

**Cytochrome:** a membrane-bound complex associated with enzymes involved in drug metabolism.

**Decimal place:** the position of a digit to the right of a decimal point.

**Dispense:** to prepare and give out medicines.

**Distribution:** of drugs, refers to the movement of drugs to and from the different tissues in the body.

**Drug interaction:** when concurrently administered drugs affect the pharmacological properties of another drug.

**Drug misuse:** abuse, maltreatment or excessive use of a drug, often resulting in addiction.

**Duty of care:** a legal and professional obligation to provide care to a patient of an acceptable standard.

**Emergency prescription:** an urgent request for a supply of a prescription-only medicine, where there is an immediate need and it is impracticable to obtain a prescription without undue delay.

**Enteral:** route of administration using the gastro-intestinal tract.

**Ethical:** pertaining to the morals or principles of doing right or wrong.

**Excretion:** of drugs, the loss of drug molecules, or their metabolites, from the body.

**Excipient:** an inert substance used as a diluent or vehicle for a drug.

**Extemporaneous preparation:** a special therapeutic preparation that is compounded and dispensed by a pharmacist for certain use, usually for a short period of time and often for a named patient.

**Formulary:** a list of drugs available to be prescribed.

**GFR:** glomerular filtration rate, measures the functioning of the kidney.

**Herbal medicine:** the use of a plant, plant extract or preparation to treat a disease.

**Idiosyncratic:** A peculiar or unusual individual reaction (to a drug).

**Liability:** an obligation or responsibility for something that one is liable for.

**Mental capacity:** an assessment of a person's ability to make a rational decision. The Mental Capacity Act 2005 provides a legal definition.

**Metabolism:** in relation to drugs, is the process by which the body chemically changes drugs administered.

**Misuse of drugs:** abuse, maltreatment or excessive use of a drug or drugs, usually considered dangerous and often resulting in addiction. These are controlled under the Misuse of Drugs Act 1971.

**Negligence:** failure to take proper care in doing something, which may breach the practitioner's duty of care.

**Non-medical prescriber:** a prescriber who is not a doctor or dentist.

**Non-proprietary:** drugs that are not protected by a trademark or patent, which anyone can produce and distribute.

**Palliative:** relieving or treating the symptoms of a disease without producing a cure.

**Parenteral:** route of administration not through the gastro-intestinal tract.

**pH:** a measure of how acidic or basic a solution is.

**Pharmacovigilance:** the process of monitoring the adverse effects, risks, and benefits of a medicine.

**Polypharmacy:** the use of a number of different drugs, by a patient who may have one or several health problems.

**Proprietary:** a drug that is made and sold under the protection of a patent or trademark.

**Recreational drugs:** a substance with pharmacological effects, taken voluntarily for pleasure or satisfaction rather than for medical purposes.

**Regulatory body:** a public authority or government agency responsible for exercising autonomous authority over some area of human activity in a regulatory or supervisory capacity.

**Reuptake:** the process by which chemicals released from neurones (neurotransmitters) are absorbed back into the neurone.

**Units:** a standard measure of the magnitude of physical quantities or dimensions (e.g. grams and metres).

**Volume of distribution:** related to drugs in the body, is a calculation of the volume of plasma that would be necessary to contain the total amount of a drug in a patient's body if the drug was present everywhere at the same concentration.

**Yellow Card Scheme:** scheme by which reports of adverse effects or interactions with drugs can be made by health professionals.

# References

Atreja, A., Bellam, N. and Levy, S.R. (2005) Strategies to enhance patient adherence: making it simple, *Medscape General Medicine*, 7(1).

Dean, B., Schachter, M., Vincent, C. and Barber, N. (2002) Causes of prescribing errors in hospital inpatients: a prospective study, *Lancet*, 359(9315): 1373–8.

Department of Health (2006) *Improving Patients' Access to Medicines: A Guide to Implementing Nurse and Pharmacist Independent Prescribing within the NHS in England*. London: Crown.

Galbraith, A., Bullock, S., Manias, E., Hunt, B. and Richards, A. (2007) *Fundamentals of Pharmacology: An Applied Approach for Nursing and Health* (2nd edn). Harlow: Pearson Education.

Garfield, S., Barber, N., Walley, P., Wilson, A. and Eliasson, L. (2009) Quality of medication use in primary care – mapping the problem, working to a solution: a systematic review of the literature, *BMC Medicine*, 7: 50.

Haynes, R.B. (2001) Interventions for helping patients to follow prescriptions for medications. *Cochrane Database of Systematic Reviews*, 2001, Issue 1.

Horne, R., Frost, S., Weinman, J., Wright, S.M., Graupner, L. and Hankins, M. (2004) Medicine in a multi-cultural society: the effect of cultural background on beliefs about medications, *Social Science and Medicine*, 59: 1307–13.

Howard, R.L., Avery, A.J., Slavenburg, S., Royal, S., Pipe, G., Lucassen, P. and Pirmohamed, M. (2007) Which drugs cause preventable admissions to hospital? A systematic review, *British Journal of Clinical Pharmacology*, 63: 136–47.

Jones, M. (1999) *Nursing Prescribing: Politics to Practice*. Oxford: Baillière-Tindall.

Jones, M. and Gough, P. (1997) Nurse prescribing – why has it taken so long?, *Nursing Standard*, 11(20): 39–42.

Leventhal, H., Meyer, D. and Nerenz, D.R. (1980) The common sense representation of illness danger, in S. Rachman (ed.) *Contributions to Medical Psychology*, Vol. 2. New York: Pergamon Press.

Maslow, A.H. (1970) *Motivation and Personality* (2nd edn). New York: Harper & Row.

Medicines and Healthcare Products Regulatory Agency (2011) *How We Regulate Medicines* [monograph on the Internet]. London: Crown. Available at: www.mhra.gov.uk/Howweregulate/Medicines/index.htm.

National Institute for Health and Clinical Excellence (NICE) (2011) Hypertension: clinical management of primary hypertension in adults [PDF]. London: NICE.

National Patient Safety Agency (2004) *Seven Steps to Patient Safety.* London: NPSA.

National Prescribing Centre (1999) Signposts for prescribing nurses – general principles of good prescribing, *Prescribing Nurse Bulletin*, 1(1): 1–4.

Nursing and Midwifery Council (2006) *Standards of Proficiency for Nurse and Midwife Prescribers*. London: NMC.

Pirmohamed, M., James, S., Meakin, S., Green, C., Scott, A.K., Walley, T.J., Farrar, K., Park, B.K. and Brekenridge, A.M. (2004) Adverse drug reactions as cause of admission to hospital: prospective analysis of 18 820 patients, *British Medical Journal*, 329(7456): 15–19.

Silverman, J., Kurtz, S. and Draper, J. (2004) *Skills for Communicating with Patients* (2nd edn). Oxford: Radcliffe.

Sims, R. and Gardiner, E. (1999) Nurse prescribing: the lawmakers, in M. Jones (ed.) *Nurse Prescribing: Politics to Practice*. London: Baillière-Tindall.

Weinstein, N.D. (1983) Reducing unrealistic optimism about illness susceptibility, *Health Psychology*, 2: 11–20.

World Health Organization (2003) *Adherence to Long-term Therapies: Evidence for Action*. Geneva: WHO. Available at: http://apps.who.int/medicinedocs/en/d/Js4883e/5.html.